Wildernes
First Aid

A Ragged Mountain Press
Pocket Guide

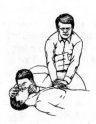 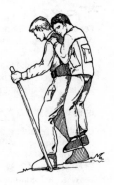

Paul G. Gill Jr., M.D.

 Ragged Mountain Press / McGraw-Hill
Camden, Maine • New York • Chicago • San Francisco • Lisbon •
London • Madrid • Mexico City • Milan • New Delhi • San Juan •
Seoul• Singapore • Sydney • Toronto

Look for these other Ragged Mountain Press Pocket Guides:

Backpacker's Pocket Guide, Chris Townsend
Edible Wild Plants and Herbs, Alan M. Cvancara
Sea Kayaker's Pocket Guide, Shelley Johnson

Ragged Mountain Press
A Division of The McGraw-Hill Companies

10 9 8 7 6 5 4 3 2 1
Copyright © 2002 Ragged Mountain Press
All rights reserved. The publisher takes no responsibility for the use of any
of the materials or methods described in this book, nor for the products
thereof. The name "Ragged Mountain Press" and the Ragged Mountain
Press logo are trademarks of The McGraw-Hill Companies. Printed in the
United States of America.

ISBN 0-07-137962-2

Questions regarding the content of this book should be addressed to
Ragged Mountain Press
P.O. Box 220
Camden, ME 04843
www.raggedmountainpress.com

Questions regarding the ordering of this book should be addressed to
The McGraw-Hill Companies
Customer Service Department
P.O. Box 547
Blacklick, OH 43004
Retail customers: 1-800-262-4729
Bookstores: 1-800-722-4726

This book is printed on 60# Thor White Antique by R. R. Donnelley
Illustrations by William Hamilton; Design by Geri Davis, Davis Associates,
and Anton Marc; Production management by Janet Robbins; Page layout
by Deborah Evans; Edited by Tom McCarthy, Jonathan Eaton, and Shana
Harrington.

NOTE: The information in this book is intended to supplement, not replace,
the medical advice of trained professionals. All health matters require medical supervision; consult your physician regarding any condition that may
require diagnosis or medical attention. Readers with chronic medical problems or a history of drug allergy, as well as all pregnant or breastfeeding
women, should consult their physicians before taking any of the medications recommended in this book. The author and publisher disclaim any
liability arising directly or indirectly from the use of this book.

For
Hampar Kelikian, M.D.
1899–1983
Surgeon, Man of Letters, Humanitarian

Contents

Spider, Scorpion, Insect, and Snake Bites and Stings

Plant Dermatitis

Infectious Diarrhea and Field Water Disinfection

Symptom Charts

Introduction

Wilderness First Aid: A Ragged Mountain Press Pocket Guide was written for all who venture into the wilderness, seeking to regain, however briefly, the sense of independence and equanimity that modern life tends to leach from us all. Kayakers, anglers, campers, backcountry trekkers, cross-country skiers, hunters, and modern-day Henry David Thoreaus on a Rocky Mountain Walden Pond will find this a useful companion when things go wrong. It is the successor to my earlier books on wilderness medicine: *Simon & Schuster's Pocket Guide to Wilderness Medicine*, which was born of the sports medicine column I wrote for *Outdoor Life* magazine from 1988 to 1995, and the *Ragged Mountain Press Pocket Guide to Wilderness Medicine & First Aid*. I know how quickly disaster can strike in a remote setting and how lonely and frightened people can feel when they suddenly find themselves disabled, in pain, and running out of daylight, warmth, and sustenance. And I know that most individuals who seek out the wilderness are self-reliant, resourceful types who would rather get themselves out of a scrape than accept help from others. And so my articles, and this book, were designed to offer sound, practical medical advice that could be used by men or women on the trail to save life or limb, using the materials they carried with them or could collect from their surroundings.

The responses of readers and book reviewers encourage me to believe that this book succeeds in its objective. Perhaps most gratifying are the many letters I have received from people all over the world, asking for additional copies of the book and telling me how it helped them deal with various wilderness medical emergencies.

How to Use This Book

Wilderness emergencies rarely come with advance warning. You may discover an unconscious hiker on the trail or find your companion shivering after falling in a cold stream. You may or may not have witnessed the accident or trauma. The approach that follows assumes nothing and therefore starts at the beginning and follows a prescribed path. In all instances, you must first evaluate, then stabilize, treat, and, if necessary, evacuate the injured or ill individual from the wilderness.

Assuming you know little or nothing of your companion's condition, the first chapter contains comprehensive instructions on diagnosing and stabilizing patients suffering from a wide range of conditions and symptoms. Use this information to determine the type and severity of the injury or illness, stabilize the patient, and guide you to additional chapters that will help you to treat specific injuries or illnesses.

Once you understand the nature of the illness or injury, turn to the appropriate later chapter. Use the diagnostic symptom charts to guide you quickly to the information you need to evaluate and treat the described injury or illness.

And remember, *primum non nocere*—"first, do no harm."

Assessing and Stabilizing the Trauma Victim

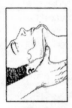

PRIMARY AND SECONDARY SURVEYS OF A PERSON WITH MULTIPLE INJURIES

THE PRIMARY SURVEY: THE ABCDEs

It is extremely important that you do not move the victim until you are certain that there is no spinal injury. (If the victim does have a fracture or a fracture-dislocation of the spine, the slightest movement can drive sharp fragments of bone into the spinal cord, resulting in permanent paralysis or death.) First do a primary survey to detect and treat quickly any immediately life-threatening injuries.

A. Airway. Establish that the victim is unresponsive. If a neck injury is possible, keep the head, neck, and trunk in a straight line as you move the victim into a supine position. Then open the airway using the *jaw-thrust technique*: put a hand on each side of the victim's face and lift the jaw up and forward *without tilting the head back.*

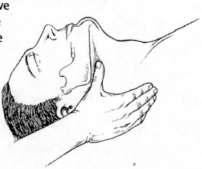

Opening the airway using the "jaw-thrust" technique.

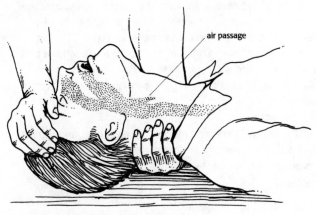

air passage

Opening the airway using the "head-tilt" technique.

If a neck injury can be ruled out, open the airway using the *head-tilt technique*: place one hand under the victim's neck and the other on the victim's forehead. Then flex the neck and extend the head.

B. Breathing. Check for breathing by watching for expansion of the chest and listening for sounds of breathing with your ear alternately near the victim's mouth and against her chest. If breathing is not detected, perform two mouth-to-mouth breaths by pinching her nostrils, taking a deep breath, sealing your lips around her mouth, and giving her two breaths of two seconds each. Then go on to C.

C. Circulation. Put your index and middle fingers over her windpipe, and slide them down alongside the neck muscle and feel for a pulse. If there isn't one, start CPR (see Cardiopulmonary Resuscitation, pages 17–18).

Then do a quick head-to-toe survey for wounds and fractures, and splint any obvious fractures (see Splints, page 40). Control bleeding by applying direct pressure to the wounds with any bulky, clean material—use your shirt if nothing else is handy. Bright red blood spurting from a wound is arterial; oozing, dark blood is probably from a vein. Arterial bleeding, especially from the scalp, neck, groin, or shoulder, can be difficult to control and can lead to the rapid, complete loss of all of the body's blood volume *(exsanguination)*. If firm pressure doesn't stop the bleeding after a few minutes, pack the wound with sterile gauze and cover it with a bulky, firmly applied bandage *(compression dressing)*. To control severe bleeding from a leg wound, push your fist into the abdomen at the level of the navel and press firmly. This compresses the aorta against the spinal column and will control the flow of blood into the legs while you apply a bulky bandage. Tourniquets are dangerous. Don't use one unless you are willing to write off the limb to save the victim.

D. Disability. Determine the victim's level of consciousness and the size and reactivity of her pupils. Use the AVPU method to evaluate her mental state.

A: *A*lert

V: responds to *V*ocal stimuli

P: responds to *P*ainful stimuli

U: *U*nresponsive

The victim's pupils should be approximately the same size and should constrict when exposed to bright light. If they aren't or don't, see Head Injuries, pages 53–55.

E. Expose. If you are sure there is no spinal injury, remove as much of the victim's clothing as necessary or advisable under the circumstances (extreme cold, etc.) so that you can inspect every inch of her body for injuries.

THE SECONDARY SURVEY

After you have attended to any life-threatening injuries, take a few minutes to examine the victim from head to toe. If it is safe to do so, roll him over so that you can do a complete exam. Use your eyes, ears, and hands to identify injuries that may have escaped your attention during the primary survey, and use this book to help you diagnose and treat the injuries you uncover.

ASSESSING AND STABILIZING THE TRAUMA VICTIM

SHOCK

IS THE VICTIM IN SHOCK?

Shock is collapse of the peripheral circulation. It can be caused by a lot of things, but in the wilderness it's usually due to bleeding (from open wounds, ruptured organs, or fractured bones); fluid loss (from heat exhaustion or snakebite); or vascular collapse secondary to insect sting.

Whatever the nature of the insult, the final result is the same: interruption of the flow of blood to the cells. The chemical reactions that power each cell are fueled by a steady flow of oxygen and nutrients in the blood. When the flow of blood is cut off, the metabolic machinery stops and the cells die.

The body's compensatory mechanisms are very efficient. A young, otherwise healthy person can lose 25 to 30 percent of his blood volume (1 to 1.8 liters of blood) and show no signs of shock other than a rapid pulse and cool, moist skin. But if the victim loses even a little more blood, shock will become progressive and irreversible. If shock is not reversed within one hour (the "Golden Hour"), the patient will die no matter what treatment is given. But shock has to be recognized before it can be treated. Here are its classic signs.

Mild shock: The victim has lost up to a liter of blood, but his body is compensating well and his blood pressure remains normal. He is alert, may complain of being cold and thirsty, and may feel weak and light-headed when he sits up. His skin is pale, cool, and damp, and his pulse is about 110 to 120 beats a minute.

Moderate shock: Blood loss is substantial, 20 to 40 percent of his volume (1 to 2.5 liters), and the victim is prostrated. He is too weak to move under his own power, his speech is slurred, and he complains of thirst and shortness of breath. His skin is cold and clammy, his pulse is very rapid and weak, and his urine output is scant.

Severe shock: The victim has lost 40 percent or more of his blood volume (2.5 liters or more), and blood flow to the heart and brain is now severely compromised. His breathing is shallow and rapid, his eyes are dull, his pupils are dilated, and he is restless and agitated and then lethargic and comatose.

TREATMENT

After you have controlled bleeding (see The Primary Survey: the ABCDEs, above), put the victim in the "shock position," with his legs flexed at the hips, his knees straight, his feet elevated 12 inches (30 cm), and his head down. This promotes the return of venous blood to the heart and enhances the flow of arterial blood to the brain.

Cover the victim with blankets or an open sleeping bag, and offer him warm fluids by mouth if he is able to swallow. Move him out of danger if you have to, but avoid rough handling. Check his pulse and breathing rate and pattern every few minutes. Remember, restlessness and agitation may be signs of worsening shock.

Make arrangements for rapid medical evacuation. Time is of the essence!

CARDIOPULMONARY RESUSCITATION (CPR)

Check for a pulse and, if absent, do chest compressions as follows.

1. Place the heel of one hand on the lower half of the breastbone, and place your other hand over the first.

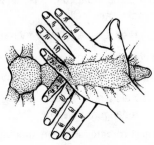

Proper hand position for chest compression.

2. Keeping your shoulders over his chest and your elbows locked, compress the chest at a rate of 100 compressions per minute, stopping every 15 compressions to open the airway and give two breaths. Depress the breastbone 1.5 to 2 inches (4 to 5 cm) with each compression.

Caution! Excessively forceful or misplaced compressions can cause fractures and injuries to internal organs. Don't let the heel of your hand slide down over the tip of the breastbone, and keep your fingers away from the chest.

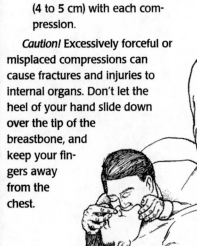

CPR.

Continue CPR until

1. breathing and pulse return

2. the rescuers are exhausted

3. the rescuers are in danger

4. the victim fails to respond to prolonged resuscitation (how you define "prolonged" depends on the circumstances; prolonged CPR is more likely to be successful in hypothermia victims)

5. the rescuers are relieved by medical professionals

Do *not* do CPR when

- the injury is lethal (death is obvious)

- rescuers would be jeopardizing their own lives by entering a dangerous setting

- chest compressions are impossible (for example, the chest is frozen or crushed)

- there is any sign of life (breathing, heart sounds, pulse, or movement)

- the victim has clearly stated, in writing, that he doesn't wish to be resuscitated

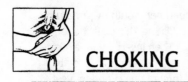

CHOKING

USING THE HEIMLICH MANEUVER

If the victim can speak, cough, or breathe, leave her alone: her airway is only *partially* obstructed. If she starts to make a high-pitched noise when she inhales, if she turns blue, or if her coughs deteriorate into feeble little grunts, the obstruction is nearly complete. If she can't talk and is clutching her throat with her hands, the obstruction *is* complete. In either case, you need to do the Heimlich maneuver.

The *Heimlich maneuver* is a series of abdominal thrusts that elevate the *diaphragm* (the breathing muscle that separates the chest and abdominal cavities), which in turn causes a sudden rise in the pressure inside the chest cavity and an artificial cough that expels the foreign object. Here is what you should do when someone is choking.

- *If the victim is standing or sitting and is conscious:* Stand behind her and wrap your arms around her waist. Place one fist thumb side in on the center of the victim's stomach just above the navel. Grab that fist with your other hand and press it into her abdomen with a quick, upward thrust. Repeat the maneuver until the airway is cleared or she loses consciousness.

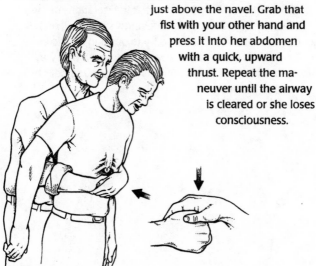

The Heimlich maneuver.

- *If the victim is unconscious:* Open her mouth by grasping the tongue and lower jaw and lifting (this pulls the tongue out of the back of the throat). Then insert the index finger of your other hand into the back of her throat and attempt to hook it behind the foreign object and move it into and then out of the mouth. (Be careful not to push the object deeper into her throat.) Then open the airway and attempt to ventilate. If you are unable to, reposition her head and try to ventilate again. If the chest does not rise, kneel astride her thighs and perform the Heimlich maneuver up to five times. Repeat this sequence as many times as needed.

- *If you are alone and choking:* Perform the Heimlich maneuver on yourself. Make a fist with one hand, and place the thumb side on the abdomen just above the navel. Grab the fist with your other hand, and press inward and upward in a quick, sharp, thrusting motion. If this doesn't work, press your abdomen across any firm surface, such as a tree stump or a rock.

A few caveats: When doing abdominal or chest thrusts, be careful not to place the fist too near the *xiphoid process* (a small piece of cartilage that projects down toward the abdomen from the breastbone) or on the lower margins of the rib cage. Fractures of the xiphoid or ribs can result in lacerations of the liver, spleen, or lungs. Also, abdominal thrusts can result in regurgitation of stomach contents, so try to position the victim so that her head is lower than the rest of her body. That way, the stomach contents will drain out of her mouth and not obstruct the airway further.

CHEST PAIN

SYMPTOMS

Insufficient blood flow *(ischemia)* to the heart muscle *(myocardium)*, usually secondary to blockage of the coronary arteries, may cause one of the following types of chest pain.

1. *Angina pectoris.* Angina is heaviness, squeezing, pressure, a choking sensation, or a vague discomfort under the sternum that lasts for 5 to 10 minutes. It may radiate to the neck, shoulders, or arms, and it is usually brought on by exertion or emotional upset and subsides with rest or nitroglycerin. However, it *may* occur at rest or during sleep and can be triggered by heavy meals, by performing unaccustomed work, or by exposure to cold.

2. *Acute myocardial infarction* (heart attack). When a blood clot or spasm of a coronary artery causes prolonged ischemia, the myocardium *infarcts* (dies). Heart attacks usually occur when the patient is at rest—most often in the morning. The patient may complain of a crushing or squeezing pain under the sternum or all across the chest and upper abdomen that radiates down the arms or into the throat, neck, back, or jaw. He may describe it as the most excruciating pain he has ever experienced, or he may try to convince you that it is just a bad case of indigestion. It may feel like a severe angina attack, but it doesn't subside with rest or after taking nitroglycerin. The patient is usually nauseated and short of breath, and he may break out in a cold sweat. His skin may be cold and clammy, his face ashen, and his lips and nail beds blue. His pulse may be rapid, irregular, and thready, and he may have a sense of impending doom.

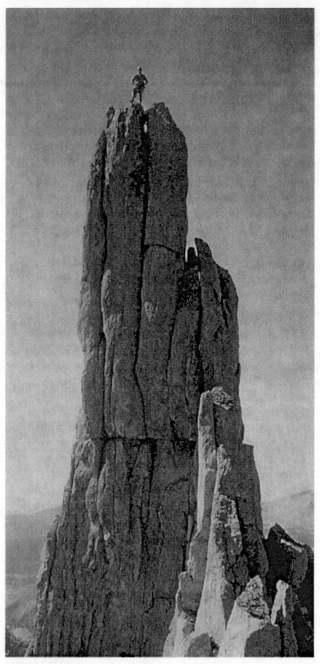

Yosemite, California

ASSESSING AND STABILIZING THE TRAUMA VICTIM

TREATMENT

Here's how you should treat someone you think is having angina pectoris or a heart attack. Place the patient in a semirecumbent position, and loosen any restrictive clothing. If you have nitroglycerin tablets, put one under his tongue. If he gets no relief, repeat every 5 minutes for a total of three tablets in 15 minutes. If he still hasn't gotten relief, he may be having a heart attack. Give him one aspirin tablet. This may limit or completely prevent heart attack damage to the heart muscle. Then do whatever you can to reassure the patient and make him comfortable while you arrange for evacuation to the nearest medical facility.

Soft Tissue Injuries

OPEN WOUNDS

CONTROLLING THE BLEEDING

Most bleeding can be controlled with firm pressure over the wound or direct pressure with your finger tips over the bleeding vessels. For severe bleeding, see The Primary Survey: the ABCDEs, pages 12–14.

CLEANING THE WOUND

After you've stopped the bleeding, the next step is to examine the wound. First wash your hands, then check to see how deep the wound is and whether there is any damage to deep structures, such as bones, nerves, tendons, and blood vessels. Remove pebbles, vegetable matter, and other foreign objects by hand, and then cleanse the wound with the cleanest water available, which in most cases will be your drinking water. Stream water is fine once the water has been disinfected (see Water Disinfection, pages 131–34). Add enough 10 percent povidone-iodine solution to make a 1 percent solution, and irrigate the wound liberally, taking pains to wash out grit, soil, and vegetable matter. Use a sterile gauze pad to wipe dirt gently out of the wound. (Scrubbing further traumatizes the tissues, increasing bleeding and risk of infection.)

The best way to dislodge small dirt particles from the wound is to inject the solution under pressure with a syringe. If

Symptom Chart: Soft Tissue Injuries

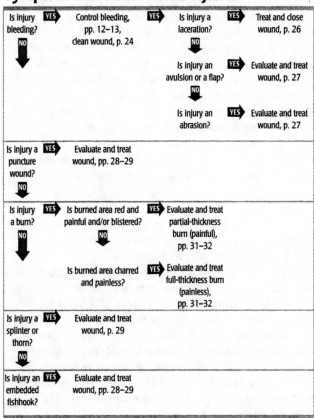

Is injury bleeding?	**YES**	Control bleeding, pp. 12–13, clean wound, p. 24	**YES**	Is injury a laceration?	**YES**	Treat and close wound, p. 26
				NO		
				Is injury an avulsion or a flap?	**YES**	Evaluate and treat wound, p. 27
				NO		
				Is injury an abrasion?	**YES**	Evaluate and treat wound, p. 27

NO ↓

| Is injury a puncture wound? | **YES** | Evaluate and treat wound, pp. 28–29 |

NO ↓

Is injury a burn?	**YES**	Is burned area red and painful and/or blistered?	**YES**	Evaluate and treat partial-thickness burn (painful), pp. 31–32
		NO ↓		
		Is burned area charred and painless?	**YES**	Evaluate and treat full-thickness burn (painless), pp. 31–32

NO ↓

| Is injury a splinter or thorn? | **YES** | Evaluate and treat wound, p. 29 |

NO ↓

| Is injury an embedded fishhook? | **YES** | Evaluate and treat wound, pp. 28–29 |

you don't have a syringe, fill a small, plastic bag with irrigating solution and poke a pinhole in the bottom. When you squeeze the bag, the solution will come out in a forceful stream. Direct the stream into the depths of the wound, under skin flaps, and at any particles that seem to be adhering to the wound. When you're done irrigating the wound, make a final inspection and remove any remaining debris.

CLOSING THE WOUND

Many wounds are best left "open" in the wilderness. No matter how meticulous you are in cleansing the wound, it is impossible to remove all contaminants from a wound when your operating theater is a clearing in the forest and your operating table is a bed of pine needles. Bacteria thrive on the blood and necrotic debris that accumulate in the depths of a contaminated wound. Closing such a wound is a recipe for wound infection. If you leave the wound open, pus can drain freely and won't accumulate to form an abscess. But each wound has to be treated according to its characteristics, including location, depth, contamination, and injury to deep structures.

It generally is safe to close facial and scalp lacerations. They rarely become infected, thanks to the rich blood supply to the head. Large scalp wounds usually have to be closed to control bleeding. The simplest way to do this is to tie clumps of hair across the wound until the bleeding stops.

Many lacerations can be closed with micropore tape. Shave excess hair, and then apply tincture of benzoin to the skin on either side of the wound to make the tape stick better (be careful not to get any in the wound itself—it stings!). Then dab a little antibiotic ointment on the wound. When the benzoin has dried, apply several tapes across the wound. The best technique is to first anchor one end of the tape to a wound edge and then pull that edge up snug to the opposite edge, making sure the wound edges are even. These tapes should stay in place until the wound has healed.

Trunk and extremity lacerations should be cleaned as well as possible, skin edges taped together, coated with antibiotic ointment, and covered with a sterile dressing in layers. The first layer should be a sterile, nonabsorbent dressing, such as Tegaderm. The next layer should be absorbent sterile pads, followed by a large surgical dressing (Surgipad) if the laceration is large and compression is needed to control bleeding. The dressings can be then be taped in place or wrapped with roller gauze.

If the wound is particularly dirty, use wet-to-dry dressings. Apply wet sterile gauze pads directly to the wound, and change them twice a day. When the dressing is dry, remove it along with crust and debris. This is an effective way to control infection in any wound.

SOFT TISSUE INJURIES

SKIN AVULSIONS AND FLAPS

When a knife or other sharp object strikes the skin at a shallow angle, it often tears off a hunk of skin. This is called an *avulsion*. Avulsions come in two forms: partial-thickness avulsions, in which just the top layers of the skin are lost, and full-thickness avulsions, in which all of the skin and possibly some of the underlying tissue are lost.

Avulsions are treated the same way as lacerations, but no attempt should be made to close an avulsion. Since skin is missing, the wound has to heal from the bottom out. All fingertip avulsions heal, providing bone isn't exposed. Exposed bone must be covered with a skin graft, and any avulsion larger than a half-dollar generally will require skin grafting.

A *flap* is an avulsion in which the skin and underlying fatty tissue are intact on one side. A flap often will survive if its blood supply is good. A pale flap has no blood supply and can be expected to turn black gradually and fall off, but it can still serve as a "biologic dressing" while the wound heals from beneath. Flaps should be cleaned gently with antiseptic solution and then bandaged. If the wound turns red and starts to drain pus, infection has set in. The flap can be lifted off to promote drainage, and wet-to-dry dressings can be applied.

ABRASIONS

An abrasion is what you get when you skin your knee or elbow or scrape the superficial layer of skin over any bony prominence, such as the front of the leg, knuckles, or chin. Dirt may be ground into these wounds, so you need to spend some time washing them, using either a mild soap or an antiseptic solution. Small abrasions can be covered with a transparent dressing, such as Bioclusive or Tegaderm adhesive dressings. These are waterproof dressings that "breathe." They keep water out but allow oxygen to penetrate to the healing tissues, and they can be left on for several days. Larger abrasions should be bandaged the same way as a laceration—with antibiotic ointment, a nonabsorbent dressing, and a few layers of absorbent gauze for compression. The dressing should be changed daily until a firm scab forms (resist the temptation to pick off the scab—it's a natural dressing).

PUNCTURE WOUNDS

The wound may not look like much, but that rusty nail, thorn, or wood splinter may have driven bacteria and dirt deep into the tissues. It also may have punctured a blood vessel, nerve, tendon, or joint lining.

TREATMENT

A puncture wound is a tetanus-prone wound. Irrigate it thoroughly with antiseptic solution; then apply antibiotic ointment and a light dressing. (Make sure your tetanus immunization is up-to-date before you leave home.)

HOW TO REMOVE EMBEDDED OBJECTS

Removing a Fishhook
The string technique:

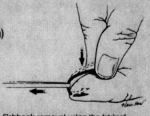

Fishhook removal using the "string" technique.

1. Loop a 12-inch (30 cm) length of string around the curve of the hook and wrap the ends around your index finger.

2. Push down on the eye and shank of the hook with your free hand to disengage the barb.

3. Align the string with the shank's long axis. Then gently tug on the free ends of the string until the barb comes out through the entrance wound.

The push-and-snip technique:

1. If the barb is protruding through the skin, snip it off and back the hook out.

2. If the barb *isn't* protruding, wash the skin around the wound with antiseptic solution; then numb it with an ice cube. Grasp the shank of the hook with a pair of

needlenose pliers or a hemostat, and push the point of the hook through the skin.

3. Snip off or flatten the barb; then back the hook out.

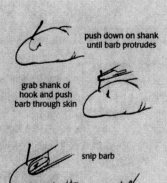

push down on shank until barb protrudes

grab shank of hook and push barb through skin

snip barb

back out hook

Fishhook removal using the "push-and-snip" technique.

Removing a Splinter or a Thorn

There are two things you should know about splinters. They are always harder to remove than you think they are going to be, and your best shot at removing a splinter is your first attempt. The more you poke at it, the more fragmented it becomes, the farther you push it into the wound, and the less cooperative will be your patient. So sit the patient and yourself down, make sure your lighting is good, and get out your finest tweezers.

Before you start, press on the skin around the entrance wound and get a feel for the orientation of the splinter under the skin. Put your finger against the point of the splinter that is embedded in the skin, and push it toward the entrance wound. Then get a good hold of the exposed portion of the thorn or splinter with your tweezers, and pull in the opposite direction to that in which it entered the skin. After you get the splinter out, wash the wound with antiseptic solution and apply antibiotic ointment and a dressing.

Large, impaled objects should be left in place, especially if they are in the eye, neck, chest, or abdomen. That arrow, stake, or what-have-you may be the only thing preventing catastrophic bleeding from a perforated blood vessel. Instead, stabilize the object by wrapping it in a bulky bandage; then evacuate the victim to a hospital.

BURNS

The size of burns is expressed in terms of the percentage of body surface burned. The easiest way to do this is to use the *rule of nines*, in which the head is considered to be 9 percent, the front and back of the torso each 18 percent, each upper extremity 9 percent, each lower extremity 18 percent, and the genitals 1 percent of the body surface area.

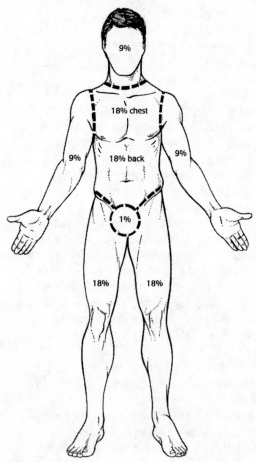

The "rule of nines."

  SOFT TISSUE INJURIES

TYPES

Partial-thickness burns: Partial-thickness (first- and second-degree) burns are red and painful and may have large blisters. If they are red and painful without blisters, they are first-degree burns. Blisters indicate that they are second-degree burns. With these burns, the hair follicles and nerve endings are undamaged and sensation is preserved. If infection is kept at bay, these burns will heal.

Full-thickness burns: Full-thickness (third-degree) burns have a charred, leathery, or waxy appearance. Ironically, since the skin is destroyed, so are its nerve endings, and full-thickness burns are virtually painless. Full-thickness burns larger than a silver dollar usually require skin grafting.

Scalds and friction burns: A pot of boiling water can be knocked off a campfire or portable stove just as easily as off the kitchen stove back home. The result is the same, of course: partial-thickness burns with large blisters or full-thickness burns. Treat them the same as any other thermal burn.

Friction, or "rope," burns can range from mild superficial abrasions to deep thermal burns and shredding of the skin of the palms of the hands or other unprotected body parts. They are treated in the same manner as other burns.

TREATMENT

Partial-thickness burns involving less than 10 percent of the body can be considered *minor* and don't require hospitalization. Apply cool compresses for a few minutes to give immediate relief of pain. Then gently clean the burn with disinfected water and mild soap or antiseptic solution, using a cotton ball to remove dirt and debris. Don't disturb intact blisters. All burns with blisters, open or closed, should be treated with a thin (⅛ in., or 3 mm) layer of triple antibiotic or silver sulfadiazine (Silvadene) cream and covered with Spenco 2nd Skin (if it is a small burn) or a fine-mesh roll gauze bandage and then bulkier dry (Kling) gauze bandage. Fingers and toes should be bandaged individually. The dressing should be carefully loosened with warm water and removed daily, and the burn washed with mild soap and then re-dressed. By changing the dressings daily, accumulated pus and necrotic debris are removed and the wound is kept clean. If you don't have any ointment or dressings, simply allow the burn to scab over. The scab will help to protect it against infection.

A partial-thickness burn will heal if it doesn't become infected. Burns are tetanus-prone, so make sure your tetanus booster is up-to-date. (*Note*: Do not apply Silvadene to the face. Use antibiotic ointment instead.)

The following types of burns are to be considered *major* burns: second-degree burns covering more than 10 percent of the body or third-degree burns over more than 5 percent of the body; most burns involving the face, eyes, ears, hands, feet, or genitals; circumferential burns; burns associated with fractures and other significant trauma; and less severe burns in anyone younger than age 5 or older than age 60. These people should be evacuated rapidly to a hospital. When the body is denuded of a significant amount of its skin, shock from fluid loss and overwhelming infection is inevitable unless fluid is replaced and the burns are covered with sterile dressings. While awaiting medical evacuation, keep the victim's extremities elevated to promote drainage, and encourage the victim to take fluids by mouth if she is alert and in no respiratory distress.

CRUSH INJURIES

CONTUSIONS

A contusion is a deep bruise, a crush injury to skin and underlying muscle. Blood vessels in the skin and muscle rupture, causing black and blue marks *(ecchymoses)* on the skin and a pool of blood in the muscle *(hematoma)*.

Treatment: Contusions and hematomas are treated the same way as strains and take about four to five days to heal. Large contusions can be quite painful and may mask serious underlying injury. A hard blow to the back can cause a contused kidney, usually manifested as blood in the urine. A severe blow to the chest can cause a contused lung, which will cause shortness of breath and coughing up of blood.

SUBUNGUAL HEMATOMAS

When you drop a rock on the end of your finger, the nail bed (the tissue under the nail) bleeds into the confined space under the nail. As pressure builds up under the nail, the nail turns blue and the pain becomes exquisite.

Treatment: The simplest remedy is to drain the hematoma with a hot paper clip. Or you can drill a hole in the nail with a knife or a needle point. (First make certain that the end of the finger isn't fractured: push down against the tip—if it is not particularly tender, it is probably not fractured.)

Musculoskeletal Problems: Bones, Joints, and Muscles

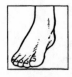 ## <u>SPRAINS</u>

A sprain is an injury to the ligaments that hold a joint together. In a mild to moderate sprain, the ligament is stretched and up to 75 percent of its fibers are torn. In a severe sprain, all or nearly all of the fibers are torn.

RICE (rest, ice, compression, and elevation) is the key to treating sprains. The objectives are to limit swelling and bleeding and to relieve pain. Swelling increases pain and prolongs healing. And the more you move the injured joint, the more it's going to bleed, so rest it.

Ice slows bleeding and deadens the sensory nerves in the injured area. (If you don't have ice, try immersion in cold water or application of a wet towel.) An elastic bandage wrapped around a sprained ankle or wrist provides compression that also prevents bleeding and swelling. Apply the ice over the bandage for 30 minutes. Then remove the ice and bandage to allow blood to flow into the injured area. After 15 minutes, reapply the elastic bandage and ice bag. Repeat this cycle several times during the first 24 to 48 hours. Also, be sure that the bandage isn't wrapped too tightly. If your toes or fingers start to hurt, tingle, or turn white or blue, remove the bandage immediately.

Keep the injured limb elevated above heart level to reduce swelling. If pain and swelling persist after 48 hours of RICE, substitute warm soaks or compresses for ice. Continue to elevate the part, and keep it wrapped in a pressure dressing or splint when it's not soaking. When the pain subsides, gradually start to use the extremity.

Symptom Chart: Musculoskeletal Problems

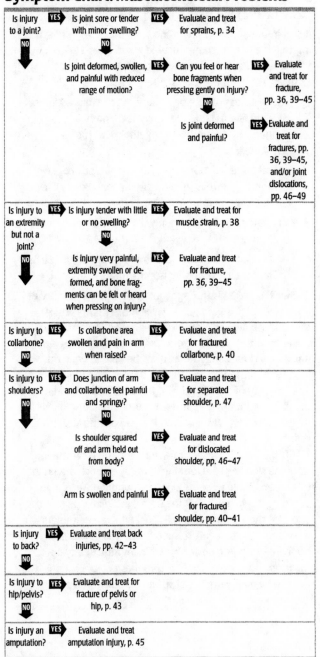

Is injury to a joint? — **NO** ↓
Is injury to a joint? — **YES** → Is joint sore or tender with minor swelling? — **YES** → Evaluate and treat for sprains, p. 34

Is joint sore or tender with minor swelling? — **NO** ↓
Is joint deformed, swollen, and painful with reduced range of motion? — **YES** → Can you feel or hear bone fragments when pressing gently on injury? — **YES** → Evaluate and treat for fracture, pp. 36, 39–45

Can you feel or hear bone fragments when pressing gently on injury? — **NO** ↓
Is joint deformed and painful? — **YES** → Evaluate and treat for fractures, pp. 36, 39–45, and/or joint dislocations, pp. 46–49

Is injury to an extremity but not a joint? — **YES** → Is injury tender with little or no swelling? — **YES** → Evaluate and treat for muscle strain, p. 38

Is injury tender with little or no swelling? — **NO** ↓
Is injury very painful, extremity swollen or deformed, and bone fragments can be felt or heard when pressing on injury? — **YES** → Evaluate and treat for fracture, pp. 36, 39–45

Is injury to an extremity but not a joint? — **NO** ↓

Is injury to collarbone? — **YES** → Is collarbone area swollen and pain in arm when raised? — **YES** → Evaluate and treat for fractured collarbone, p. 40

Is injury to collarbone? — **NO** ↓

Is injury to shoulders? — **YES** → Does junction of arm and collarbone feel painful and springy? — **YES** → Evaluate and treat for separated shoulder, p. 47

Does junction of arm and collarbone feel painful and springy? — **NO** ↓
Is shoulder squared off and arm held out from body? — **YES** → Evaluate and treat for dislocated shoulder, pp. 46–47

Is shoulder squared off and arm held out from body? — **NO** ↓
Arm is swollen and painful — **YES** → Evaluate and treat for fractured shoulder, pp. 40–41

Is injury to shoulders? — **NO** ↓

Is injury to back? — **YES** → Evaluate and treat back injuries, pp. 42–43

Is injury to back? — **NO** ↓

Is injury to hip/pelvis? — **YES** → Evaluate and treat for fracture of pelvis or hip, p. 43

Is injury to hip/pelvis? — **NO** ↓

Is injury an amputation? — **YES** → Evaluate and treat amputation injury, p. 45

IS IT FRACTURED?

If you injure an extremity in the wilderness, you are going to have to make an educated guess as to whether you are dealing with a broken bone or a lesser injury. Here are some tip-offs to fractures.

- Gently press on the bones around the injured joint. If there is a fracture, you may feel and hear the bone fragments rubbing together. This is called *crepitus.*

- A fractured wrist or finger will look deformed, unless the fracture is hairline. If your wrist looks like an upside-down fork, it is broken.

- If the joint is dislocated, it will usually be even more deformed.

- If the victim can move the limb through a full range of motion, it's probably not fractured.

Swelling alone is not a reliable guide to the severity of an injury. Sprains sometimes swell more than fractures. You can usually walk, although with pain, on a sprained ankle or foot. If the thin bone on the outside of the ankle (the *fibula*) is broken, you may still be able to walk on that leg because the fibula is not a weight-bearing bone. The majority of ankle and foot fractures, though, are too painful to walk on. If your wrist is broken, your grip will be weak. You won't be able to hold a walking stick in that hand.

Check the skin over the fracture. If bone is protruding from the skin, you are looking at an open fracture. Put the cleanest possible dressing on the wound before you do anything else. Then splint the limb (see Splints, page 40), and give the victim cefadroxil (Duricef), 1 gram immediately and 500 mg every 12 hours. There is a danger of bone infection *(osteomyelitis)* and gangrene in any open fracture, and people who develop these complications have to be evacuated to a hospital as quickly as possible.

WRISTS, HANDS, FINGERS, AND TOES

Wrist injuries should be immobilized in a *cock-up splint*. Put a rolled-up pair of socks in the palm of the hand, and rest the wrist and hand on a 10-inch-long (25 cm) piece of cardboard or wooden slat. Then wrap an elastic bandage around the hand from the knuckles to 6 inches (15 cm) above the wrist.

The cock-up splint keeps the wrist in a natural, comfortable position and prevents the hand from getting stiff. It's also the best way to immobilize a sprained or badly bruised hand. (*Warning*: There is no way to tell if a wrist is fractured without X-rays. As soon as you get home, have your doctor look at it. An untreated wrist fracture can result in permanent loss of function of the hand and chronic pain and disability.)

Use the buddy system for sprained fingers and toes. Tape the injured digit to its partner. Then ice and elevate it.

STRAINS

Strains are muscle injuries. Muscles can be "pulled," meaning that the muscle contracts so forcefully during a sudden movement that either it rips the tendon out of the bone or the muscle rips away from the tendon. Or the muscle itself can tear. Strains are as painful as sprains and take about as long to heal. Not surprisingly, the treatment is almost the same: RICE for 24 to 72 hours, followed by range-of-motion exercises in warm water *(hydrotherapy)* three times a day. The warm water relaxes the muscle and promotes circulation of nutrient-carrying blood to the healing tissues. Continue hydrotherapy until you have regained full, pain-free use of the muscle.

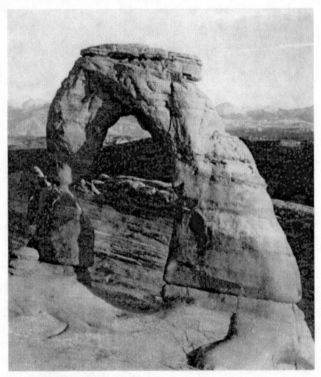

Delicate Arch, Arches National Park, Utah

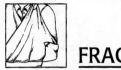

FRACTURES

CHECKING THE CMS

A fracture is a soft tissue injury complicated by a broken bone. The first step in treating a fracture in the wild is to check the circulation, motor function, and sensation (CMS) of the limb distal to (beyond) the fracture site. How you handle an injured extremity depends primarily on the results of this initial exam. If you find a loss of motor power, sensation, or circulation in the limb, this means that the bone ends are pressing on the vessels or nerves at the fracture site and that gangrene or permanent paralysis could result if you don't remedy the situation. Here's how to do a CMS exam.

Circulation: Gently remove the boot and sock if the lower extremity is injured—or the glove or mitten if the upper extremity—and feel for pulses. Feel at the wrist on the thumb side, right behind the inner knob of the ankle, or on the top of the foot between the first and second *metatarsals* (long bones), as appropriate. Then check the warmth and color of the fingers or toes. They should be pink. If they are blue or pale and cold, the circulation is impaired.

Motion: Ask the victim to wiggle his fingers or toes and to flex and extend his wrist or ankle.

Sensation: Check for perception of light touch, pressure, and pinprick.

REDUCING AND STABILIZING THE FRACTURE

If the bones are bent at an odd angle, you need to bring them back into alignment. Here is why it's important to "set" or reduce an obvious fracture.

- to relieve the pressure of bone ends pressing on nerves and blood vessels
- to stop bleeding at the fracture site
- to prevent a closed fracture from becoming an open fracture

- to relieve pain
- to be able to apply a splint to the limb

After stabilizing the fracture, you will have to make a decision regarding evacuation. Some fractures can be definitively treated in the field. Others will be angulated and will require reduction under anesthesia. Reduction of uncomplicated fractures can be put off for up to seven days without jeopardizing the final result. But anyone with an open fracture or a fracture associated with significant blood loss, spinal cord injury, or nerve or circulatory impairment must be evacuated quickly.

SPLINTS

You can't apply a cast, obviously, but you *can* effectively immobilize most fractures with splints made from rope, brush and tree branches, metal pack frames, pack straps, sleeping pads, and maps. On a long trek, you'd be smart to bring along a selection of wire or pneumatic or padded aluminum splints. Splinting the fracture in the functional position will decrease bleeding and damage to soft tissues, prevent stiffness, and make the victim more comfortable. The splint should immobilize the joint above and the joint below the fracture and should provide some compression, but not so much that it cuts off the circulation. Loosen any compressive bandages or wraps every two hours to check CMS, and don't forget the RICE (see page 34).

TYPES

Clavicle fractures: Fractures of the *clavicle* (collarbone) are usually obvious. After a fall onto the shoulder, you'll have swelling and crepitus over the middle of the collarbone and pain on upward movement of the arm. Treatment consists simply of wearing a sling for 10 to 14 days or until you feel comfortable without it. If you don't have sling material, simply position the arm across the lower chest and secure the sleeve in position with safety pins. If the victim is wearing a short-sleeved shirt, pull the bottom edge of the shirt up and over the forearm and then pin it to the sleeve and chest portion of the shirt with safety pins.

Shoulder fractures: A hard fall on the side or back of the shoulder can crack the *humerus* (upper arm bone) near the shoulder. There will be marked swelling and pain in the arm.

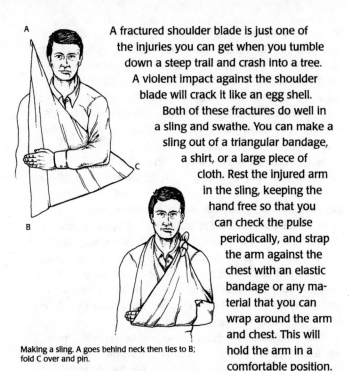

A fractured shoulder blade is just one of the injuries you can get when you tumble down a steep trail and crash into a tree. A violent impact against the shoulder blade will crack it like an egg shell.

Both of these fractures do well in a sling and swathe. You can make a sling out of a triangular bandage, a shirt, or a large piece of cloth. Rest the injured arm in the sling, keeping the hand free so that you can check the pulse periodically, and strap the arm against the chest with an elastic bandage or any material that you can wrap around the arm and chest. This will hold the arm in a comfortable position.

Making a sling. A goes behind neck then ties to B; fold C over and pin.

Upper arm fractures: Fractures of the mid- to upper arm are unstable fractures, and muscle forces cause the fracture to bow forward. A common complication of mid-humerus fractures is *wrist drop*, the inability to extend the wrist or fingers due to pressure on the radial nerve that supplies the wrist and finger extensor muscles.

Immobilize these fractures by firmly applying wood slats or similar materials to both the inner and the outer aspects of the upper arm and securing them with an elastic bandage. Then put the arm in a sling and swathe. If there is a wrist drop, splint the wrist in a position of function with a cock-up splint (see page 37).

Elbow fractures: The elbow doesn't have much padding. If you slip on a rock and land on your elbow, it's not the rock that will crack. Immobilize fractures of the elbow in a sling with the elbow flexed to a right angle.

Forearm fractures: Fractures of both bones in the forearm are unstable and should be firmly splinted and then put in a sling. If the forearm is badly deformed and CMS is impaired, take hold of the arm by the wrist and apply steady, gentle traction.

When the arm looks straight, splint it and put it in a sling. Sure, it'll hurt a little. But reducing the fracture will do wonders for the circulation to the arm and hand, and your buddy will be much more comfortable when his fractured wing is splinted and resting in a sling. Be sure to check the CMS of the fingers at regular intervals after you reduce the fracture. Loosen the splint if the pulse is weak, if there is any loss of motion or sensation in the fingers, or if the fingers turn blue or white.

Wrist fractures: If, after a fall on the outstretched hand, the wrist looks like an upside-down fork, the wrist is fractured. But one of the small bones could be fractured and not produce a deformity. If there is any question of a fracture, make a cock-up splint, as described under Sprains on page 37. (This is also a good way to splint a sprained or badly contused hand.) If you can't find a pulse at the wrist, or the fingers are cold and blue, you may be dealing with a fracture-dislocation. Reduce it by grasping the victim's hand in yours, handshake fashion, and pull straight out until the deformity is corrected. Check the circulation, and then splint as described above.

Hand fractures: Fractures of the long bones of the hand are usually stable and require nothing more than an elastic bandage or a cock-up splint (see page 37). Reduce angulated fractures of the fingers by pulling straight out on the injured digit. Splint the finger with an aluminum splint or by taping it to the adjoining finger (known as a *buddy splint*).

Crushed fingertips should be thoroughly cleaned, dressed, and then protected with a short splint applied to the last third of the finger.

Lumbar spine fractures: Most back injuries are due to twisting, bending, or lifting movements that injure the muscles, ligaments, and discs of the lower *(lumbar)* spine. These generally respond to a day or two of rest, along with warm compresses and analgesics.

Falling off a cliff never hurt anyone, but those hard landings will get you every time. Rapid deceleration produces tremendous compression forces, which can crush the vertebral bodies, usually in the midback area. A severe injury will result in fracture-dislocation of the spine. In a situation like this, you have to assume that the spinal cord is injured until you find evidence to the contrary (see pages 51–52). If the victim has to be moved, logroll him to avoid further injury to the spinal cord. Then do a quick neurologic exam: Check his grasp strength;

then ask him to wiggle his toes and bend his knees and hips. Check to see whether he can feel light touch, pressure, and pinprick over the arms, legs, and trunk. If his motor strength and sensation are normal, roll him onto one side and check for fractures by gently thumping over the entire spinal column. If you find a tender area, you can assume that there is a compression fracture at that level. Gently roll him back onto his back, check for other injuries, and arrange for medical evacuation. If the neurologic exam is normal and you don't find any tender areas in the spine, you can assume that there is no serious spinal injury and tend to his other injuries.

Pelvis, hip, and thigh fractures: Fractures of the hip, pelvis, and thigh bone *(femur)* are potential killers. You can easily lose a quart of blood from one of these fractures. Pelvic fractures are frequently multiple and can result in massive blood loss, shock, and tears in the bladder. Such injuries in the wilderness will challenge your resourcefulness and will. Here is how to handle them. If a fractured pelvis or hip is suspected and weight bearing is painful, place the victim in a supine position. If she complains of pain in the groin and the leg appears shorter than the other and is rotated outward, she probably has a fractured hip. Splint the fracture by strapping the legs together. Make a litter or sled, put her on it, and head for home. (A roll under the knees will make her a little more comfortable during the trip.) Stop periodically and check for signs of shock: pale, cool, wet skin; rapid, thready pulse; and agitation.

Fractures of the shaft and lower end of the femur are more problematic. Powerful muscles attach to this bone, and spasm of these muscles causes the sharp bone ends to pierce muscle and other soft tissues, causing heavy bleeding. These fractures must be immobilized immediately. If there are extra hands available, have one person apply steady traction to the leg by pulling on the foot while another person applies countertraction to the pelvis. Pull until the pain is relieved (this will usually require a force of about 10 percent of the victim's body weight), and maintain traction on the leg while a splint is being applied. One simple splinting technique is to secure the broken leg to the uninjured one. Or you can strap a tree branch, a paddle, or some other long object to the leg from chest to ankle, but make sure there is padding over all bony prominences, including the knee and ankle. Put a soft roll under the knee so

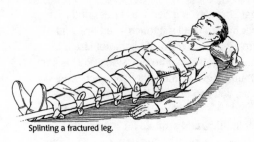

that the knee is flexed about 5 or 10 degrees.

If there are six or more people in your party, you can consider transporting the vic-

Splinting a fractured leg.

tim out overland. If you don't have the manpower, send someone for a rescue crew.

Kneecap fractures: The kneecap is another of those un-padded bones. A fractured kneecap *(patella)* can be hard to distinguish from a bad bruise. If there is a lot of swelling over the front of the knee and you feel crepitus when you press down on the kneecap, it's probably broken. The best treatment is a cylindrical splint from groin to ankle. A rolled-up foam sleeping pad will do nicely. Climbing will be almost impossible with this injury, but the victim can walk over gentle terrain with the help of a walking stick.

Lower leg fractures: A fall from a height may result in a fracture of the upper part of the leg bone *(tibia)*. Such fractures usually involve the knee joint, and bleeding will cause the knee to swell like a balloon. Fractures of the shaft of the tibia are frequently angulated and open, and the thin bone that runs alongside the tibia (the *fibula*) is usually broken also. If the leg is deformed and CMS is impaired, realign the bones by grasping the ankle and applying steady traction along the long axis of the bone until it straightens out. Then splint it. If the bone is protruding, wash the fracture site with antiseptic solution (or soap and water), and apply a sterile dressing or the cleanest cloth bandage available. Then reduce and splint the fracture. If you have antibiotics in your medical kit, give the victim cefadroxil as directed on page 36.

Ankle fractures: Ankle fractures and sprains are often nearly indistinguishable: a swollen, tender ankle could as easily be fractured as sprained. Run your fingers over the bony knob on each side of the ankle, feeling for deformity and crepitus. If you find none, call it a sprain and apply the RICE technique, as described on page 34. If ice isn't available, cold water or snow will help to reduce swelling and alleviate pain.

The victim may be able to walk with some help. If there is no deformity, it may be better to leave his boot on. It will make an excellent splint, and you'll never get it back on once it has been off for a while.

Fractures of the ankle are often associated with dislocations. These are usually obvious, with the foot discolored and bent at a weird angle. This puts the stretch on the blood vessels in the area, and prompt reduction is necessary to save the foot. Stand or kneel facing the bottom of your patient's foot. Then grasp the foot, with the heel in one hand and the other hand over the top of the foot, and pull steadily toward you. The ankle will slip back into place with a "thud," and a nice pink color will return to the foot as the circulation returns. A pillow, down parka, or other soft, bulky object wrapped around the ankle and pinned in place makes an excellent splint.

Foot fractures: Jumping from a height and landing on the feet is a recipe for a fractured heel or long bone of the foot (*metatarsal*). Fractures of the heel are often associated with compression fractures of the spine, so make sure that you examine that area also. Splint suspected fractures of the heel area as you would an ankle fracture. A stiff-soled boot makes a good splint for metatarsal fractures.

Fractured toes heal nicely if you just tape them to their buddies. Put a little cotton between the toes to absorb moisture and prevent skin maceration. There is a great deal of pressure on the big toe during the toe-off phase of walking, so fractures of this digit can be disabling. Stiff-soled boots help to take some pressure off the fracture, especially if you tape four or five tongue depressors across the sole at its widest part.

AMPUTATIONS

Amputations are treated the same way as an open fracture (see page 36). Control bleeding by holding firm pressure over the stump with a bandage or rolled-up clothing. Then irrigate the stump with disinfected water before applying a sterile dressing secured with an elastic bandage. The amputated part should be cleaned and transported with the victim. Cover it with a moistened, sterile bandage, and put it in a plastic bag, filled with ice if possible.

DISLOCATIONS

Reducing a dislocated joint can be like trying to put Jack back in the box. It's a tough job, but someone has to do it—and quickly. If you don't pop that shoulder (or elbow, finger, or hip) back in right away, swelling and muscle spasm will make the job next to impossible. And reducing the dislocation provides instant pain relief, takes the pressure off the nerves and blood vessels around the joint, and allows you to splint the injured limb in a comfortable position.

A wound over a dislocated joint constitutes an *open disloca-tion*. Joint infection is a serious threat. Clean the wound thor-oughly and apply a sterile bandage before attempting to reduce it. *Always* check CMS before and after reduction (see page 39), and start the patient on cefadroxil, 1 gram immedi-ately and 500 mg every 12 hours.

TYPES

Here are some of the common dislocations encountered in the wilderness and how to handle them.

Dislocated shoulder: Dislocated shoulders are common in-juries and are relatively easy to reduce. They are usually the re-sult of a backward force on an elevated arm. *Warning*: Before you start yanking on that "dislocated" shoulder, make sure that it really is out of joint. If you don't have X-ray glasses, this can be tricky. But you can be reasonably sure of your diagnosis if

- the shoulder has an unnatural, "squared-off" appearance
- the arm is held out from the body
- the victim can't place her hand on the uninjured shoulder

Here is one way to reduce a dislocated shoulder. Have the victim lie prone on a ledge or other flat surface with the dislo-cated arm hanging over the edge. Use strips of cloth or other material to secure a weight of 10 to 15 pounds (4.5 to 7 kg) to the wrist. Then take a short hike. When you return in 10 min-utes, the shoulder will be back in joint.

Here is another technique. Position the victim as before, with the injured arm hanging over an edge. Sit or kneel next to her, wrap your hands around her upper arm, and gently pull down on the upper arm. Gradually increase the downward

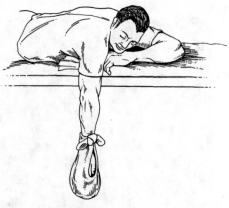

Reducing a dislocated shoulder.

force on the arm until you feel the shoulder slip back into joint. You'll know when it's back in when you hear the victim give a huge sigh of relief and a beatific smile spreads across her face.

Immediately after reducing the shoulder, put the arm in a sling and swathe, keeping the hand and wrist free so that you can check the circulation at regular intervals.

Separated shoulder: One common error is to mistake a "separated" shoulder for a dislocation. A *separation* generally is caused by a fall directly onto the shoulder, causing disruption of the ligaments that connect the collarbone with the shoulder blade *(scapula)*. In a partial separation, the ligaments are only partially torn, and you will find swelling and tenderness over the end of the collarbone. In a complete separation, the ligaments are totally disrupted, and the end of the collarbone appears to be elevated an inch (2.5 cm) or more. (You can distinguish between a separation and a fractured collarbone by pressing over the end of the collarbone. If it feels "springy," you are dealing with a separation. If the collarbone is very tender and feels "crunchy," it's fractured.) Separated shoulders should be immobilized in a sling.

Dislocated elbow: You will know a dislocated elbow when you see one. A hard fall on the arm drives the forearm bones backward and out of the elbow joint. These dislocations can be tough to reduce, but it's worth a try if you are more than a few hours from help. Pull slowly and steadily on the forearm while an assistant pulls in the opposite direction on the upper arm. You will feel the elbow go back in, and the victim will be able to bend it to 90 degrees.

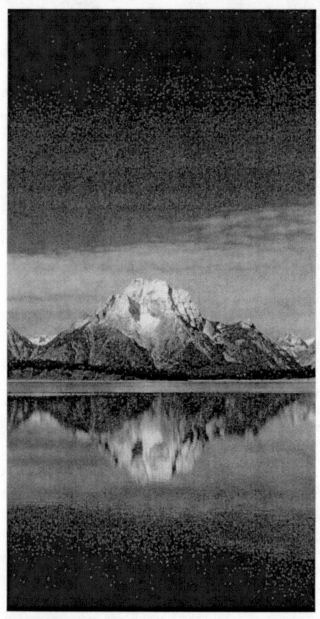

Grand Teton National Park, Wyoming

If one or two good efforts fail to reduce the dislocation, put the arm in a sling and hit the trail. Undue force will only result in unnecessary pain and damage to the joint, nerves, and blood vessels.

Dislocated finger: Dislocations of the first joint of the finger are common on wilderness treks, usually the result of the finger being struck and bent back by a thrown object. A dislocated finger is always obvious. Reduce it by pulling straight out on the deformed digit with one hand while pushing the base of the dislocated bone back into joint with the thumb of your other hand. Then splint the finger to its buddy.

Dislocated hip: It takes a fall off a cliff or a similar violent injury to dislocate the hip, a very stable "ball-and-socket" joint. Either the thigh will be sticking out at an odd angle *(anterior dislocation)* or the leg will be shortened, rotated inward, and crossed over the uninjured leg *(posterior dislocation)*.

While reducing a dislocated hip in the wild is no mean feat, it should be attempted. The longer the hip is out of socket, the greater the risk of complications, including damage to the sciatic nerve and necrosis of the ball part of the joint. Lay the victim supine on the ground, and slowly bend the knee and hip to 90 degrees so that the knee and foot are pointing up. Have an assistant push down on the hips while you straddle the victim, place his leg between your thighs, and wrap your hands behind his knee. Then pull up hard on his thigh while you gently rotate the leg first one way and then the other. When you feel the hip go in, splint it to the other leg with soft padding between the knees. If you cannot reduce it, splint it in a comfortable position and arrange to evacuate the victim.

Dislocated kneecap: Scrambling down a rocky mountainside can cause a sudden twisting motion of the knee, which can dislocate the kneecap. A direct blow to the inner side of the kneecap will do the trick too. The kneecap will be displaced laterally, and the knee will be flexed 45 or 60 degrees. These dislocations can easily be reduced by slowly straightening the knee. You may have to gently nudge the kneecap back into place by pressing laterally on it with your hand. After it's reduced, apply a cylindrical splint to keep the knee in a fully straightened position. Walking may be a little painful, but it is safe.

Head and Neck Injuries

APPROACHING THE HEAD- OR NECK-INJURED PATIENT

ASSESS THE ABCDEs AND MENTAL STATUS

The approach to the badly injured person has got to be streamlined and efficient. Start with the ABCDEs: *a*irway, *b*reathing, *c*irculation, *d*isability, and *e*xpose, as described on pages 12–14. Once you have attended to any immediately life-threatening problems, assess the victim's mental status by evaluating the following areas.

1. *Eye opening.* Does she open her eyes spontaneously or only on command or in response to a painful stimulus?

2. *Verbal response.* Is her speech understandable, and does she make sense? Or is she confused and disoriented or talking gibberish?

3. *Motor response.* Does she obey simple commands? Does she withdraw from a painful stimulus?

Then check her pupils. They should be symmetrical and re-act to light by constricting. Confusion, lethargy, garbled speech, and unequal or unreactive pupils are all signs of possible brain injury.

The next step is to resuscitate the trauma victim with the materials at hand. She might need oxygen, intravenous fluids, blood transfusion, antibiotics, and a urinary catheter, but if it's just you and her on a rocky crag, you're not going to be able to do much more than make her comfortable and perhaps give her a drink of water. (*Warning:* If she has a serious head injury, fluids by mouth are out because she could aspirate them into her lungs.)

Symptom Chart: Head and Neck Injuries

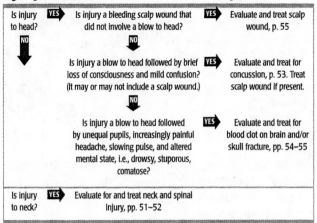

Is injury to head? **YES** → Is injury a bleeding scalp wound that did not involve a blow to head? **YES** → Evaluate and treat scalp wound, p. 55

NO

Is injury a blow to head followed by brief loss of consciousness and mild confusion? (It may or may not include a scalp wound.) **YES** → Evaluate and treat for concussion, p. 53. Treat scalp wound if present.

NO

Is injury a blow to head followed by unequal pupils, increasingly painful headache, slowing pulse, and altered mental state, i.e., drowsy, stuporous, comatose? **YES** → Evaluate and treat for blood clot on brain and/or skull fracture, pp. 54–55

Is injury to neck? **YES** → Evaluate for and treat neck and spinal injury, pp. 51–52

CERVICAL, THORACIC, AND LUMBAR SPINE FRACTURES AND LOW BACK STRAIN

Most back injuries are due to twisting, bending, or lifting movements that injure the muscles, ligaments, and discs of the lower *(lumbar)* spine. These generally respond to analgesics and warm compresses. As you do your head-to-toe exam, check for signs of spinal fractures. Remember, any blow to the head, face, or neck or any fall from a significant height can produce a spinal injury. The golden rule of spinal injuries is that every trauma victim has one until proved otherwise. If he does have a fracture or fracture-dislocation of the spine, the slightest movement can drive sharp fragments of bone into the spinal cord, resulting in permanent paralysis or death.

Ask the victim if he has pain in his neck or back. Then, without moving him, run your fingers down his spinal column from the base of the skull to the base of spine, feeling for tenderness or any abnormal prominence. If there is any sign of a neck injury, immobilize the neck by applying "sandbags" (sacks stuffed with dirt or tightly bundled clothing) around his neck, head, and shoulders. The sandbags can then be anchored in place with rocks, or a strip of adhesive tape can be drawn across his forehead and secured to the bags on either side. If you suspect a back injury, keep the victim in a supine position.

After immobilizing the spine, look for a *spinal cord injury*. Remember that children, and sometimes adults, can have a spinal cord injury in the absence of a spinal fracture or dislocation, and it's possible to

Immobilizing the neck.

have a spinal fracture but no spinal cord injury. These are the signs of a spinal cord injury.

- pain in the neck or back radiating down the arms or legs
- numbness or tingling in the hands or feet
- loss of sensation in the arms or legs
- paralysis of the arms or legs
- a sustained penile erection *(priapism)*

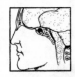

HEAD INJURIES

With head injuries, what you see is not always what you get. It's hard not to get excited when your partner hits her head on a rock overhang and lays her scalp open down to the bone. The bleeding can be horrendous, and she may turn pale and feel punk for awhile. But that doesn't mean that she has a brain injury. On the other hand, she could have serious bleeding *inside* her skull with nary a mark on her scalp. Of far greater importance than the appearance of the scalp is her mental state. Was she knocked unconscious? Is she awake and alert now? Is she oriented to her surroundings, or does she think she's on the planet Tralfalmador? Check her orientation to person, place, and time. Then decide whether she has one of the following injuries.

CONCUSSION

You don't have to be a neurosurgeon to treat most brain injuries in the wild. That's because most of these injuries are simple concussions. A *concussion* is a transient disturbance of brain function following a blow to the head. The hallmark of a concussion is a brief loss of consciousness, often followed by a period of mild confusion, memory loss, headache, and perhaps some nausea and vomiting. These symptoms resolve within a few hours or days at the most.

INTRACRANIAL BLEEDING

You *do* have to be a neurosurgeon to treat a blood clot on the brain *(subdural* or *epidural hematoma)*. Any blow to the head, especially over the relatively thin part of the skull just above the ear, can cause a tear in the vessels in or under the covering of the brain (the *dura*). Because the skull is a rigid compartment, there's no room for expansion. So when a vessel on the surface of the brain bleeds, it forms a clot that increases the pressure within the skull. When the pressure becomes great enough, blood flow to the brain ceases and the brain dies. It's "thanks for the memories" at this point, unless something is done to relieve the pressure. That means immediate evacuation to a hospital (see Wilderness Evacuation, page 147).

A person who develops a blood clot on the brain may be knocked

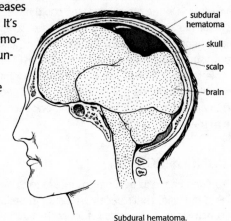

Subdural hematoma.

unconscious and never regain consciousness. Or he may regain consciousness for a brief period (the "lucid interval") only to lapse back into unconsciousness. Occasionally (especially in older people) there is no initial loss of consciousness, but increasing confusion and lethargy progressing to coma occur some hours or days after the injury.

How do you know when your partner has a life-threatening clot on the brain? Unless there's a CT scanner there in the woods, you won't know. You're going to have to keep a close eye on him for at least 24 hours, observing for

- personality changes
- vomiting

- increasing headache
- unequal pupils (if one pupil becomes as big as a saucer, he has a very serious problem: the brain is being squeezed out of the skull, and the situation is desperate)
- dropping pulse rate (as the pressure in the head rises, the blood pressure goes up and the heart rate slows)
- blood or clear fluid draining from the ears or nose (this may be a sign of a fracture of the base of the skull)
- obvious fracture or indentation of the skull (run your fingers through the hair, feeling for fractures, depressed areas, and lacerations)
- bruises behind the ears and "raccoon eyes" (also signs of a fractured skull)
- spinal injury (15 percent of victims of severe head injury also have a broken neck; if the victim is unconscious, assume he has a broken neck and immobilize his head)

REPAIRING A SCALP WOUND

Scalp wounds can bleed like Old Faithful. The best way to control the bleeding is to sew them up. If you don't have the wherewithal, here's an alternative that doesn't require needle and thread: Clean the wound, irrigating it with the cleanest water available, and pick out dirt particles, sticks, and so on. Then moisten the hair on either side of the laceration and twist small clumps of hair into braids all along the wound edges. Tie these braids across the wound until it's closed up tight. Then apply a turban dressing with a few rolls of gauze or cloth. The wound will have to be explored and closed under sterile conditions later, but this technique will control bleeding in the meantime. (*Warning*: If there is an obvious skull fracture, *don't* irrigate the wound. That would only drive dirt and bacteria into the brain. Just apply a sterile dressing and a bulky bandage. If there is an arrow, rock, or other foreign object embedded in the skull, *don't touch it!* Doing so could result in catastrophic bleeding into the brain. Apply a bandage to the wound with the object in place.)

EVACUATION

When do you evacuate the head injury victim? You can best make this judgment by assigning her to one of three risk groups.

1. *Low risk.* The victim has sustained a mild blow to the head but was not rendered unconscious, and she complains only of minor headache and dizziness. She may have a small laceration or bruise on the scalp, but her pupils are symmetrical and she has no sign of neurologic injury.

2. *Moderate risk.* The victim has had a brief loss of consciousness, vomiting, persistent or worsening headache, and amnesia for the events immediately following the injury.

3. *High risk.* The victim was knocked unconscious and now has a depressed level of consciousness or loss of sensation or strength on one side of the body. Anyone who has fallen more than 15 feet (4.6 m), has sustained a high-energy blow from a falling rock or other object, or has suffered a skull fracture or a penetrating injury to the skull should be considered at high risk, even if there was no loss of consciousness or there is no other sign of brain injury.

MAKING A DECISION

Someone who falls into the low-risk group can be expected to do well but should be watched carefully for 24 hours. She will need to be evacuated if she develops signs of lethargy, drowsiness, personality change, forceful or persistent vomiting, or abnormal gait or speech. Someone in the high-risk category must be evacuated as quickly as possible. The disposition of someone in the moderate-risk group depends on a number of factors, including other injuries and evacuation time. Generally, anyone in this group who also has spinal or other injuries should be evacuated at once.

As for the person with a neck or back injury, if he has only minimal pain and there's no paralysis, he can safely walk out under his own power. If he has significant pain but no sign of a spinal cord injury, keep him immobilized and recheck him every 20 minutes. Subtle signs of spinal cord injury may become apparent only after repeated exams. If there are *definite* signs of a spinal cord injury, go for help. Any attempt to move the victim at this point can result in catastrophe.

Evacuating an unconscious person from the wilderness can be a daunting challenge, so hit the trail while the victim is still awake and able to cooperate in his evacuation. If he is alert, he can walk without assistance. But keep a close eye on him, especially when going over rough terrain that may require normal balance and judgment.

If you have enough strong people in your party, it may be best to evacuate an unconscious person yourselves. But make sure that the victim's neck is rigidly immobilized if there is any possibility of spinal injury. Carry him supine on a litter with his head slightly elevated. If he vomits, lower his head and turn him on his side so that he doesn't aspirate the vomited material into his lungs. (If his spine is immobilized, logroll him onto his side.) Make sure that you put padding under his shoulders, elbows, buttocks, and heels to prevent pressure sores.

Chest and Abdominal Injuries

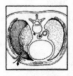

CHEST INJURIES

EVALUATING THE INJURY

The chest is a bellows, a device that by alternate expansion and contraction draws air into and out of the lungs. When the chest muscles and diaphragm contract, the chest expands, creating negative pressure in the chest cavity. Air rushes into the lungs for a few seconds and then is expelled as the chest muscles relax. Any injury that violates the integrity of the chest wall or causes an obstruction of the respiratory tree will make breathing difficult or impossible, and then it's "curtains for certain," unless you intervene to set things right.

You'll have to rely on your senses of sight, touch, and hearing to evaluate a chest injury in the wild. Physical diagnosis is based on the examiner's ability to inspect, feel, percuss, and listen for signs of disease or injury. Here's how to examine the chest.

1. *Inspect.* First make sure that the victim has an adequate airway and that she is breathing. Count the number of breaths per minute, and note the breathing pattern. The normal breathing rate at rest is 12 to 20 breaths a minute. Very slow, fast, or irregular breathing denotes trouble. How is her color? If she's blue, she's not breathing effectively. Look at the neck. Are the veins distended? That may be a sign of a tension pneumothorax (see below). Is the *trachea* (windpipe) in the center of the neck or pushed over to one side (another sign of tension pneumothorax)? Expose the chest and look for abrasions, lacerations, puncture wounds, or asymmetrical movement.

2. *Feel.* Gently run your hands over the chest, from the collarbones to the abdomen and from the breastbone to the backbone. Note any tender areas, signifying broken or con-

Symptom Chart: Chest and Abdominal Injuries

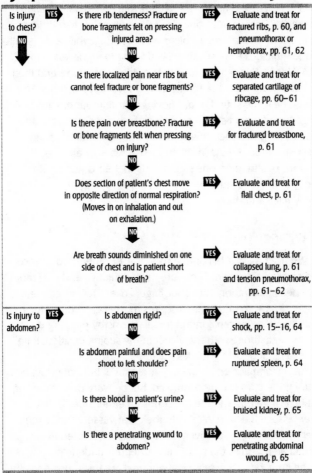

Is injury to chest? **YES**	Is there rib tenderness? Fracture or bone fragments felt on pressing injured area? **YES**	Evaluate and treat for fractured ribs, p. 60, and pneumothorax or hemothorax, pp. 61, 62
NO ↓	**NO** ↓	
	Is there localized pain near ribs but cannot feel fracture or bone fragments? **YES**	Evaluate and treat for separated cartilage of ribcage, pp. 60–61
	NO ↓	
	Is there pain over breastbone? Fracture or bone fragments felt when pressing on injury? **YES**	Evaluate and treat for fractured breastbone, p. 61
	NO ↓	
	Does section of patient's chest move in opposite direction of normal respiration? (Moves in on inhalation and out on exhalation.) **YES**	Evaluate and treat for flail chest, p. 61
	NO ↓	
	Are breath sounds diminished on one side of chest and is patient short of breath? **YES**	Evaluate and treat for collapsed lung, p. 61 and tension pneumothorax, pp. 61–62
Is injury to abdomen? **YES**	Is abdomen rigid? **YES**	Evaluate and treat for shock, pp. 15–16, 64
	NO ↓	
	Is abdomen painful and does pain shoot to left shoulder? **YES**	Evaluate and treat for ruptured spleen, p. 64
	NO ↓	
	Is there blood in patient's urine? **YES**	Evaluate and treat for bruised kidney, p. 65
	NO ↓	
	Is there a penetrating wound to abdomen? **YES**	Evaluate and treat for penetrating abdominal wound, p. 65

tused ribs or breastbone. If there is a crunchy feeling over the bone, it's probably fractured. A bubbly feeling under the skin *(subcutaneous crepitus)* is a sure sign of a collapsed lung. What you're feeling is air that has leaked out of the lung and passed into the tissues under the skin. You might feel crepitus anywhere from the neck to the groin.

3. *Percuss.* Place your long finger at various points on the chest wall, and tap the end of it with the long finger of your other hand. You should hear a slightly hollow sound from the

collarbones to about the sixth rib in the front, and from the shoulder blades to about the tenth ribs in the back. Is there a marked difference from one side to the other? A very hollow percussion note indicates collapse of the lung, while a very dull sound indicates a chest cavity filled with blood *(hemothorax)*.

4. *Listen.* Put your ear to first one side of the chest and then the other, and have the victim take several deep breaths. You should hear the sound of air moving into and out of each lung. A loud, harsh sound on one or both sides indicates obstruction of the upper airway. A wheezing or rattling sound suggests blood or fluid in the bronchial tubes or air sacs. The absence of sound on one side means that air is not moving into that lung, because of either a collapsed lung or a chest cavity filled with blood.

TYPES

Rib fractures: A fall onto a rock, log, or other hard surface can crack a rib or two. These are painful injuries and hurt more with deep inspiration. Run your fingers over the injured area. A tender area with underlying crepitus most likely represents a fractured rib. You can confirm the diagnosis by pressing down on the breastbone with the victim in the supine position. If he complains of pain in a rib, it's fractured.

An uncomplicated rib fracture is a painful but not disabling injury if the pain can be controlled. But be wary of fractures of the first three ribs and the lower ribs on either side. They are often associated with injuries to the great vessels and to the liver and spleen, respectively. Also, multiple fractured ribs should alert you to the possibility of serious underlying injury to the lung, heart, vessels, or abdominal organs. A person with this type of injury needs to be evacuated.

Treatment: The victim will need to take aspirin or a narcotic analgesic for a few days. You can stabilize the fracture somewhat by wrapping a large elastic bandage around the victim's chest. Remind the victim to take a few deep breaths every once in a while to reduce the risk of pneumonia developing in underaerated lung segments under the fracture.

Separated cartilage: Rather than joining directly to the breastbone, the ribs connect to a short segment of cartilage, which then joins the breastbone. A hard blow to the front of the chest can cause a disruption of this rib–cartilage junction *(separated cartilage)*. This type of injury is very painful and is hard to distinguish from fractured ribs.

Treatment: Treatment is the same as that for fractured ribs.

Fractured breastbone: It's not easy to break the breastbone. It requires the kind of high-energy impact you'd get from falling off a cliff. In this type of injury, there will be tenderness and crepitus over the breastbone and the chest may have a caved-in appearance. This is a serious injury and is often associated with contusions of the heart and lacerations of the lung.

Treatment: Attend to the ABCDEs (see pages 12–14), and arrange for rapid medical evacuation. The victim will be able to breathe more easily in an upright position (this is true of any chest injury).

Flail chest: Three or more consecutive ribs fractured in two or more places constitute an unstable segment of chest wall, or *flail chest*. You can diagnose this injury by looking for paradoxical movement of the chest wall in the area of the injury. When the rest of the chest is expanding, the negative pressure in the chest cavity will pull in on the "floating" flail segment, and positive pressure will cause it to move outward with expiration. Obviously, this interferes with normal breathing. The lung tissue under the flail segment is often contused or lacerated. Classically, this type of injury is tolerated fairly well for a day or two, and then the victim goes into respiratory failure, often requiring artificial ventilation for a while.

Treatment: Give the victim analgesics, and evacuate him before he deteriorates.

Pneumothorax (collapsed lung): When air enters the chest cavity through a hole in the chest wall, or a fractured rib pokes a hole in the lung, pressure rises in the chest cavity until the lung collapses. This is a *pneumothorax*. The victim will be short of breath, breath sounds will be diminished on the affected side, and you'll hear a hollow sound when you percuss over the collapsed lung. This is a painful injury, but she may be able to walk out of the woods under her own power.

Treatment: All but small pneumothoraces require insertion of a chest tube to drain air from the chest cavity. You won't be doing this in the wilderness.

Tension pneumothorax: When air leaks from a punctured lung into the chest cavity but can't escape, that side of the chest will fill up with air. The pressure increases to the point that the heart, great vessels, windpipe, and other midline structures are pushed over to the opposite side of the chest. The great veins in the chest become kinked, and venous blood can't return to the heart. The victim turns blue, the neck veins become engorged, and cardiovascular collapse ensues. This is called a *tension pneumothorax*.

Treatment: Death is imminent if the chest isn't decompressed immediately. (*Warning*: This technique requires a large, sterile needle and proper training.) The needle is inserted into the space between the second and third ribs at any point lateral to the nipple. Guide the needle over the top of the third rib and then perpendicularly down into the chest until you hear a gush of air as the needle enters the chest cavity. The victim's appearance will improve dramatically after this procedure, but he's still not out of the woods. Leave the needle in place, and make arrangements for a hasty evacuation to a hospital, where a chest tube can be inserted.

Hemothorax: Rib fractures can cause bleeding from the artery that runs along the undersurface of the rib or from a punctured lung. The blood collects in the chest cavity, causing a *hemothorax*. The victim will be in a lot of pain and short of breath. If you tap over the affected side, it will sound dull. An isolated hemothorax is not an immediate life-threatening injury. Blood loss into the chest cavity is rarely enough to cause shock, and respiratory distress is usually not severe.

Treatment: There's nothing you can do for the victim except to make her as comfortable as possible while awaiting evacuation.

Penetrating chest wounds: A hole in your chest can ruin your whole day. Backpackers have been known to transfix themselves on ski poles, ice axes, and tent poles. This is serious business. Even if the offending object misses the heart, lungs, and great vessels (an unlikely proposition), at the very least it's going to poke a hole in the chest wall and create a pneumothorax or *hemopneumothorax* (air and blood in the pleural cavity). If it punctures the chest below the nipple line, there's an excellent chance that it will skewer the liver, spleen, or other abdominal organs.

In the old movie Westerns, they'd just yank the arrow out of the guy's chest and he'd be all set to return to the action. That's *not* the thing to do. The impaling object has created a channel through the tissues. As long as it occupies that channel, bleeding will be controlled by the *tamponading* (compressing) effect it has on torn blood vessels. Always leave the arrow, pole, or what-have-you exactly where it is.

One of the most dangerous chest wounds is the *sucking chest wound*. If the hole in the chest wall approaches the diameter of the windpipe, it becomes impossible for the bellows mechanism to create negative pressure in the chest cavity, and the lungs won't expand. Instead, air is sucked through the hole in the chest into the chest cavity. It's like trying to run a vacuum cleaner when there's a large hole in the canister.

Treatment: You have to act fast when confronted with a sucking chest wound. Cover it with the cleanest bandage available—a shirt, a towel, or even your hand, if necessary. After the victim is stabilized, you can take the time to apply a sterile, petrolatum gauze dressing (Adaptic, for example) right over the wound and cover it with a sterile 4-by-4-inch (10 by 10 cm) gauze pad. Tape the pad on three sides so that air can escape but not enter through the wound. (If you seal the wound up tight, you'll create a tension pneumothorax.) As with any chest wound, the victim must be evacuated ASAP.

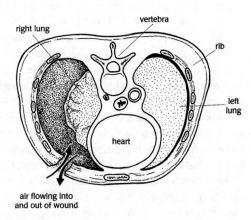

Sucking chest wound.

ABDOMINAL INJURIES

BLUNT ABDOMINAL INJURIES

Blunt abdominal injuries are rarely as dramatic or immediately life-threatening as chest injuries, but they can be just as deadly. It's rare for a chest injury to lead to hemorrhagic shock. However, you can easily lose a couple of quarts of blood from a ruptured spleen or liver. As blood collects in the rigid chest cavity, the pressure within the cavity increases until the bleeding vessels are *tamponaded* (compressed). But as blood collects in the abdominal cavity, the abdominal wall stretches and a lot of blood can be lost before pressure rises within the cavity.

Blunt abdominal injuries are rarely obvious. The key is to know when to look for these injuries and then to examine the victim carefully at regular intervals. Obviously, if your partner slips and falls belly down on a tree stump, you're going to think about blunt abdominal trauma. But you should also think about blunt abdominal trauma if he cracks his breastbone or a few lower ribs. Pain in the abdomen referred to the left shoulder should alert you to a ruptured spleen.

First, look for signs of shock: thready pulse, blue fingertips, agitation, rapid breathing, and cold, clammy skin. Then, if you have no reason to suspect a spinal injury, gently roll him onto his back and expose his abdomen. Note any bruises or discoloration, and check for rib fractures. Is his belly soft, or are his muscles rigid? Gently press under the rib cage on the right (liver) and left (spleen), the pit of the stomach, and both lower quadrants. A bruised abdominal wall may cause localized tenderness, but if you find persistent rigidity and tenderness, along with signs of shock, you've got to assume that he has a blunt injury. Treat him like any shock victim, and prepare to evacuate him. (A swollen, tight abdominal wall is a very late sign of abdominal bleeding and will be accompanied by signs of late shock.)

A blow to the flank or the back can injure the kidneys. The hallmark of a contused or ruptured kidney is blood in the urine *(hematuria)*. If the kidney is just contused, the hematuria will stop within a few hours. If the kidney is lacerated or ruptured, it may continue to bleed, causing persistent hematuria and, eventually, signs of shock. Treat the shock, and prepare to evacuate the victim.

PENETRATING ABDOMINAL INJURIES

You don't have to be a surgeon to diagnose a penetrating abdominal injury. There are usually plenty of clues. These are the important things to keep in mind.

- Any wound from the nipple line to the groin can involve the abdominal contents.

- If bowel is protruding through the wound, *don't push it back in!* Stool will soil the abdominal cavity, causing peritonitis. Just cover eviscerated bowel with moist dressings.

- These injuries need prompt surgical exploration and repair. Apply sterile dressings to all wounds, and evacuate the victim as quickly as possible.

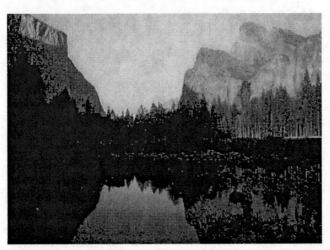

Yosemite, California

Eye, Ear, and Nose Problems

EYE INJURIES

CORNEAL FOREIGN BODIES AND ABRASIONS

These are the most common eye injuries in the wild. The *cornea* is the clear membrane that overlies the iris, the colored part of the eye. It's the most sensitive structure in the body. When the wind blows a grain of sand in your eye, it can feel like a boulder. It will make your eyes water and your lids snap shut like the jaws of a bear trap. Most often, tears will wash out sand and other foreign bodies. That's the good news. The bad news is that they are sometimes caught under the upper lid and are dragged back and forth across the cornea a few times before they are washed away, leaving you with a painful corneal abrasion. The important thing to know about a corneal abrasion is that it feels *exactly* like a corneal foreign body.

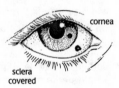

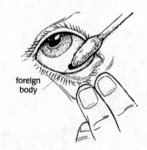

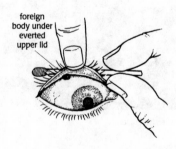

Removing a foreign body from the eye.

Symptom Chart: Eye, Ear, and Nose Problems

Is injury to eye(s)? **YES**	Is injury a small foreign body in eye? **YES**	Evaluate and treat for foreign body in eye and/or corneal abrasion, pp. 66–67
NO	**NO**	
	Is injury an object embedded in eye? **YES**	Evaluate and treat injury, pp. 67, 68
	NO	
	Is injury a cut, puncture, or contusion to eye? **YES**	Evaluate and treat for blunt or penetrating eye injury, p. 68
	NO	
	Is vision blurry and eye burns after bright day with snow and ice on ground? **YES**	Evaluate and treat for snow blindness, p. 69
	NO	
	Is vision blurry and eyes red following exposure to cold strong winds? **YES**	Evaluate and treat for frozen cornea, p. 69
Is injury to ear? **YES**	Does ear feel full with yellow soupy discharge? **YES**	Evaluate and treat for swimmer's ear, p. 70
NO	**NO**	
	Is there loss of hearing and blood oozing from ear following injury? **YES**	Evaluate and treat for ruptured eardrum, pp. 70–71
Is injury to nose? **YES**	Is bleeding present from nostrils? **YES**	Evaluate and treat for nosebleed, p. 71

Here is what you do if sand, grit, or embers blow into your eye: Have your partner take a good look at the eye. She should first check the shape and symmetry of the pupils and do a rough vision check (she should ask you to count fingers or read newsprint). Then she should search carefully for foreign bodies, checking the cornea, under both lids, and in the corners. (Use a cotton swab or a match stem to invert the upper lid, a common hiding place for grit.) If she sees something, she should try to flush it out with a gentle stream of clean water. If that doesn't do it, pull the upper lid down over the lashes of the lower lid. Or she can use a cotton swab or the corner of a piece of cloth to lift a piece of sand off the cornea.

If the pain persists, you probably have a corneal abrasion. Avoid bright light and bear with it for 24 hours. If the eye is still painful after 24 hours, there may be a small particle embedded in the cornea. It will have to be removed by a physician as soon as possible.

BLUNT AND PENETRATING EYE INJURIES

The eye is set back in a protective bony casement, but swinging branches and flying rocks can inflict devastating damage. Lacerations, puncture wounds, and contusions are usually obvious. A *hyphema* is bleeding in the front chamber of the eye, just behind the cornea. It can lead to glaucoma and blood staining of the cornea. Fluid in the back chamber of the eye seeping through a tear in the retina causes the thin retina to peel off the back of the eye like loose wallpaper. This is known as a *detached retina*. A *dislocated lens* is usually pushed backward, but you may see it in the front chamber of the eye.

These are all severe, vision-threatening injuries. There is not much you can do about them except to gently wash dirt and debris away from the eye with disinfected, warm water, cover *both* eyes with opaque eye shields (to minimize eye movement), and evacuate the victim to the nearest medical facility. *Never* attempt to remove a foreign body that is embedded inside the eyeball. If a fishhook, thorn, or some other large object is embedded in the eye, do *not* attempt to remove it. Prevent further damage by taping a paper cup over the eye; then evacuate to the nearest hospital.

SNOW BLINDNESS AND FROZEN CORNEA

Snow blindness is sunburn of the corneas. You're more likely to get it at high altitudes, where ultraviolet radiation (UVR) is more intense (4 percent increase in intensity for each 984-foot, or 300-meter, gain in altitude) and where snow and ice reflect up to 85 percent of incident UVR into your eyes. UVR in the UVB range (280–320 nanometers) is absorbed by the thin layer of cells on the surface of the cornea. (UVA is transmitted to the lens, where it can cause cataracts over time.) These cells swell and rupture, and the cornea becomes hazy. You won't realize what's going on for 6 to 12 hours. Then your eyes will begin to water and redden, your lids will swell, and you'll feel as though you have hot cinders in your eyes.

Snow blindness is temporary, and the corneas heal spontaneously in about 24 hours. But there are some things you can do to relieve the pain. First remove contact lenses. Then apply cold compresses to the eyes, and take an analgesic. Avoid the problem altogether by wearing sunglasses. If you forget your sunglasses, you can fashion a crude pair by cutting narrow slits in cardboard or some other material and strapping it to your head with string or elastic.

Frozen cornea is a windchill injury. You can get it by trying to force your eyes open while walking into a stiff breeze on a very cold day. The symptoms are similar to those of a corneal injury or snow blindness: blurred vision, lid spasm, sensitivity to light, and red, watery eyes. There is no pain, however, until the corneas start to rewarm. Treatment consists of rapid rewarming with warm (104°F, or 40°C) compresses.

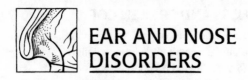

EAR AND NOSE DISORDERS

SWIMMER'S EAR

Swimmer's ear *(otitis externa)* is a bacterial infection of the outer ear canal. It is common during the summer months because heat and constant moisture break down the natural barriers to infection in the inner part of the external ear canal. Swimming, frequent showers, and mechanical trauma all predispose to infection with *Streptococcus* and *Pseudomonas* bacteria. Swimmer's ear can cause a sense of fullness in the ear, diminished hearing, intense earache, and a soupy yellow-white discharge. Pulling on the ear lobe causes intense pain.

Treatment: Carefully irrigate the ear canal with sterile or potable water; use a bulb syringe or even a cup. Instill several drops of vinegar or Burow's solution four times day. You can avoid swimmer's ear by keeping the ears dry, by not using ear plugs or cotton swabs, and by instilling a little vinegar and rubbing alcohol in the ears after each swim or shower.

RUPTURED EARDRUM

It's not hard to get poked in the ear with a branch while working your way through dense underbrush. If the branch perforates the eardrum, you will have sudden, intense pain in the ear, vertigo, hearing loss, and bleeding from the ear. The branch may have damaged the small bones *(ossicles)* in the middle ear, so the ear should be examined by a physician as soon as possible.

If you get smacked in the ear by a swinging branch and notice a loss of hearing as well as bleeding from the ear, the eardrum is probably perforated. In these situations, the eardrum usually heals nicely if left alone. Never put *anything* in the ear if a perforated eardrum is suspected.

A blow to the ear can cause a pool of blood *(hematoma)* to collect under the skin of the auricle. A large hematoma will lead to "cauliflower ear" if it is not drained. Cleanse the skin with antiseptic solution; then insert a sterile needle into the center of the hematoma and drain as much of the blood as possible. Then apply a compression bandage and an ice bag to the ear.

INSECTS IN THE EAR

Few things are as maddening as the feel and sound of an insect crawling around inside your ear. Resist the temptation to squash the bug with a cotton swab. That just creates a mess and can lead to a ruptured ear drum. Instead, take the kinder, gentler approach, and have your partner flush the critter out with warm water.

NOSEBLEED

Most nosebleeds will stop if you have the patient sit up, lean forward, and squeeze the soft part of her nose for 10 to 15 minutes. If that doesn't work, have her clear her nose. Then use a penlight to try to identify the bleeding site. Usually it will be in *Kiesselbach's area*, an area in the front part of the septum where there is a rich supply of blood vessels. Once you have found the bleeding site, cauterize it with a silver nitrate stick. If blood is draining down the back of the throat and you can't find a bleeding site, the victim may have a *posterior* nose bleed. She'll need to be evacuated to a hospital.

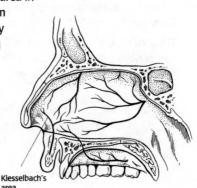

Kiesselbach's area

Hypothermia and Frostbite

THE COLD FACTS

HOW HEAT IS LOST FROM THE BODY

Whether you are hiking the Appalachian Trail in a spring downpour or are stranded in a snowstorm on a Rocky Mountain peak, your body is going to be under siege from the cold. It will mount a feverish struggle to preserve warmth, but once your core temperature drops below 95°F (35°C), you're hypothermic. Then you are on a slippery slope, and it's only a matter of time before your body's caloric reserve is depleted, your internal organs shut down, and your heart stops beating.

Actually, there is no such thing as "cold." What we perceive as cold is merely the absence of heat. But it is convenient to think of cold as a kind of magnet that pulls the heat out of your body through the following mechanisms.

- *Conduction:* the direct transfer of heat from the body to a cooler object. Normally not a major mechanism of heat loss, it is *the* major cause of heat loss during cold water immersion.

- *Convection:* the loss of heat by circulation of the air or liquid in which the body is immersed. Movement of the medium breaks up the thin layer of warm particles on the surface of the body. A fan cools by convection, and wind chill plays a big role in cooling on windy days.

- *Radiation:* the loss of heat through emitted energy. It normally accounts for over half of the body's heat loss.

- *Evaporation:* heat lost when sweat or water on the body's surface is changed into steam. Approximately 580 calories of heat are lost for each gram of water that evaporates from the skin. Perspiration increases evaporative heat loss, as does wet clothing on a windy day.

Symptom Chart: Hypothermia and Frostbite

Is patient presently shivering with possible signs of clumsiness and slurred speech? **YES** ▶	Evaluate and treat for mild hypothermia, pp. 75–76	
NO ↓		
Was patient shivering but has now stopped? **YES** ▶	Is skin cold to touch and patient responds to pain; reflexes present? **YES** ▶	Evaluate and treat for moderate hypothermia, pp. 75–76
NO ↓		
Is injury a small, whitish patch on skin after exposure to cold? **YES** ▶	Evaluate and treat for frostnip, pp. 83–84	
NO ↓		
Is the skin cold, numb, pale, or gray? Are there blisters? **YES** ▶	Evaluate and treat for frostbite, pp. 83–84	

HOW THE BODY RESPONDS TO HEAT LOSS

Humans are warm-blooded animals. We keep our internal temperature right around 98.6°F (37°C). We even have a thermostat, a part of the brain called the *thermoregulatory center*. When "cold" signals arrive from the millions of thermal sensors in the skin and elsewhere in the body, the thermostat, acting through the sympathetic nervous system, does a number of things to increase heat production and decrease heat loss.

- The muscles start to shiver, increasing heat production fivefold. Vigorous exercise increases heat production by 1000 percent.

- Blood vessels in the skin and limbs constrict. This limits radiant heat loss from the body surface, but even more importantly, it preserves the flow of warm blood to a core of vital organs (brain, heart, lungs, and digestive organs) and shunts blood from the cold shell of skin, muscle, and fat.

- The heart beats faster and harder.

- Sweating stops, decreasing evaporative heat loss.

- The metabolic rate increases up to sixfold, increasing the heat generated by the chemical reactions in each cell.

The body's furious response to the cold is like turning on your car heater when you're stranded somewhere. It's great while it lasts, but sooner or later you're going to run out of gas. When that happens, the situation deteriorates in a hurry. Eventually, the muscles become too tired and too energy starved to shiver. They become stiff and sluggish when the body's core temperature drops below 90°F (32.2°C), and the heart and metabolism slow, fluid shifts out of the circulation into the spaces between the cells, fluid is lost through the kidneys, and the blood pressure drops. With further cooling, the brain becomes sluggish, and the heart becomes irritable. Below 80°F (26.7°C), you become stiff and unresponsive and have no detectable pulses. You may mistakenly be declared dead.

PREDISPOSING CAUSES

Here are some of the things that can help to turn you into Frosty the Snowman.

- *Exposure to the elements.* You can become hypothermic in the Yukon Territory just about any day, and you can become hypothermic in Georgia or anywhere else when the conditions are right. That means cool temperatures (not necessarily below freezing), high wind, and low humidity.

- *Cold water immersion.* Water is a much greater heat conductor than air, and you'll cool at least 100 times faster in water than in air at the same temperature. This effect is compounded by movement and exposure of areas of high heat loss, such as the head, neck, and face.

- *Immobility.* A fracture or other disabling injury is a double whammy: not only does it interfere with one of your first lines of defense against hypothermia (increased muscle activity and shivering), it also makes it harder for you to get out of the cold.

- *Drugs and alcohol.* Alcohol and cold are compatible—if you are a lizard. Lizards and other cold-blooded creatures don't have to worry about a thermostat. They just go with the flow. Alcohol screws up the thermostat, inhibits shivering, impairs judgment, and dilates the blood vessels in the skin. Those Saint Bernard dogs they used to send out with the whiskey barrel around their necks always came back alone.

HYPOTHERMIA

RECOGNIZING HYPOTHERMIA

To diagnose hypothermia, you have to think of it. If your partner has been buried under an avalanche, you are going to be thinking about it. If he's been hiking on a wet, blustery day, you may not. But you should always be thinking "hypothermia" whenever one of the predisposing factors is in play.

The most reliable sign of *mild hypothermia* (core temperature 93.2° to 96.8°F, or 34° to 36°C) is shivering. But you also must be sensitive to some of the more subtle signs, such as thick or slurred speech, confusion, difficulty keeping up with the group, and poor coordination. The victim of mild hypothermia may have trouble zipping his fly or hammering tent stakes into the ground, and his skin may be cool to the touch.

The person who has been shivering but has stopped and now is confused and indifferent to his surroundings has *moderate hypothermia*. His core temperature is between 86° and 93.2°F (30°–34°C), and his skin is cold to the touch and pale or blue. He's forgetful and neglects to cover up from the cold, leaving his jacket unzipped and his mittens and hat off. He may even undress or make other dangerous errors in judgment. He may become apathetic or stuporous, and he is clumsy.

If he becomes *severely hypothermic* (core temperature falls below 86°F, or 30°C), he loses all voluntary motion and reflexes and does not respond to pain. His blood pressure plummets, his pulse slows, and he is at great risk for *ventricular fibrillation* (rapid, chaotic heart rhythm). The lowest core temperature recorded in an accidental hypothermia survivor is 60.8°F (16°C).

TREATMENT

First get the victim out of the elements, remove his wet clothing, and limit further heat loss. Cover up his head and neck, and make sure he's not in contact with the cold ground.

Next estimate the severity of his hypothermia. (This is critical. If you try rewarming the victim of severe hypothermia in the field, you may kill him.) If he is suffering from mild or moderate hypothermia, give him dry clothing and put him in a sleeping bag, alone or with someone else. Or throw a blanket around him and let him sit by the fire. Hot toddies are out, but you can give him a hot drink and some high-carbohydrate food.

The victim of severe hypothermia has to be handled the same way you'd handle an angry porcupine: *very gently*. The heart becomes irritable when it's cold. Physical exertion can cause cold, acidic blood in the cold shell to surge into the heart, causing it to fibrillate. Get him out of the elements, but don't let him move around. Gently place him in a sleeping bag or under a blanket with one or two other people (with his chest in contact with his rescuers' chests) while you arrange for evacuation.

If evacuation isn't feasible, rewarm him in the field, using the radiant heat from a fire, chemical "hot packs," hot water bottles, or warmed stones or other objects. Hot baths are not a good idea for the victim of severe hypothermia. They cause the blood vessels in the skin and extremities to dilate and fill with warm blood from the core. The blood volume is already compromised by loss of fluid into the tissues and from the kidneys, so this leads to *rewarming shock*. When the cold blood returns to the heart, it can cause a paradoxical temperature "afterdrop" and fibrillation.

CPR and hypothermia: The hypothermia victim may be stiff, unresponsive, and pale and may have fixed and dilated pupils. But he is not dead until he is warm and dead. Do CPR unless he has a lethal injury, his chest is frozen, he is breathing or moving, or doing CPR would put his rescuers in danger.

Don't do CPR if his core temperature is below 82.4°F (28°C) and equal to the ambient temperature, if he's been immersed in water for more than 50 minutes, or if you are more than four hours from a hospital.

PREVENTION: DRESS FOR SUCCESS

Your body is a heat-generating machine. If you are physically fit, you will be able to maintain your body heat longer on the trail and you'll have a better chance of getting to shelter if the weather turns nasty. Get yourself into shape with a good conditioning program before you answer the call of the wild in winter.

Drink plenty of fluids when you are outside in the cold. Your metabolic furnace cannot run at full capacity if you are dehydrated. Dehydration also increases the risk of frostbite. You should also keep that metabolic furnace stoked with plenty of calories, especially the carbohydrate variety. Make sure you bring some snacks along with you on the trail.

Clothing can dramatically decrease conductive and convective heat losses. Air is a great insulator, so the key is to maintain multiple layers of warm air around your body by wearing multiple layers of clothing, which you can shed or add to as weather conditions change. The last thing you want to do is sweat excessively. That accelerates evaporative heat loss. You can doff hat and gloves when you start to feel warm and then loosen up your collar or take off your jacket and one or two underlayers as conditions dictate.

The best cold weather materials are wool, down, foam, Orlon, Dacron, polyester, Gore-Tex, Thinsulate, taslanized nylon, and Flectalon. Cotton wets easily, and its "wicking" action causes rapid cooling. You'd survive longer stark naked than you would in wet cotton in the cold.

Your cold weather wardrobe might look something like this: wool underwear (or try polypropylene, Capilene, or Olefin underwear if you anticipate working up a sweat); wool pants and shirts; wool sweater; a jacket or vest filled with down, Quallofil, or some other lofting material and having a two-way zipper; a hooded nylon or Gore-Tex parka or windbreaker; windproof and water-repellent wind pants; two pairs of socks (polypropylene and wool); a wool stocking cap or balaclava; wool or wool-lined polypropylene mittens with nylon or Gore-Tex shells; and rubber-soled, leather climbing boots or double winter mountaineering boots. Select boots with thick soles and insoles to impede conductive heat loss through the feet and plenty of toe room. Tight boots cut off the circulation to the toes and leave no room for a layer of insulating air between socks and uppers.

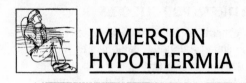

IMMERSION HYPOTHERMIA

THE COLD, HARD FACTS

Water doesn't have to have ice floes in it to qualify as "cold water." You can become hypothermic in 77°F (25°C) water. Most American rivers and lakes are cooler than that year-round.

There is a common misconception that falling into frigid water is tantamount to instant death. Actually, that's rare. The fact is, you can survive for hours in 50° to 60°F (10° to 15.6°C) water, depending on your body type and other factors. The body's core temperature remains stable for 15 minutes in cold water—time enough to save yourself, if you know what to do.

Here's what happens when you fall into cold water.

1. The cold water on your skin stimulates the respiratory center in the brain, causing you to gasp and then hyper-ventilate for a minute or two. Hyperventilation diminishes your breath-holding capacity to 15 to 25 seconds.

2. The blood vessels in your skin and muscles constrict, shutting off blood flow to the periphery and forming a cold "shell" insulating a warm "core." Your movements become sluggish.

3. You begin to shiver. Shivering is the body's main defense against hypothermia in air, but in water it's a mixed blessing. It increases metabolic heat production, but it also increases the flow of water between skin and clothing, accelerating convective heat loss.

4. As your core temperature drops below 90°F (32.2°C), you stop shivering, you become confused, and your judgment becomes impaired.

HOW LONG WILL YOU LAST
IN COLD WATER?

Because of its greater thermal conductivity and specific heat, you cool 100 times faster in water than in air at the same temperature. But not everyone who goes into the drink cools at the same rate. How fast a person cools depends on several factors.

- *Body fat.* The fatter you are, the slower you cool in water.

- *Body type.* Big people cool slower than smaller people.

- *Physical fitness.* Cardiovascular fitness helps you to handle the stress of cold water immersion, but fit people have less subcutaneous fat for insulation.

- *Water temperature.* The colder the water, the faster you cool.

- *Clothing.* Conventional thermal clothing, designed to take advantage of the insulating effect of pockets of air trapped between skin and garment, is of little value in water. These air pockets are history as soon as you hit the drink.

- *Alcohol.* If you are drunk, you are more apt to fall into cold water. In that case, you're more likely to drown than die of hypothermia.

- *Behavior.* Swimming and treading water increase the flow of warm blood from the body's core to the muscles, breaking down the "shell" insulation and increasing the cooling rate 35 to 50 percent. Exercise also accelerates cooling by increasing the flow of cold water under protective clothing.

GETTING OUT OF THE DRINK

If you go into the drink, get out of the water if you can. If
you have a boat,
pull yourself as far
out of the water as
possible. Try to
conserve energy
and body heat,
and exercise as lit-
tle as possible.
Avoid the open
body position in
the water, cover
the sides of the
chest and groin,
and go into the
HELP (*h*eat *e*scape
*l*essening *p*osture) position.

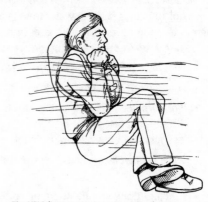

The HELP (*h*eat *e*scape *l*essening *p*osture) position.

The best way to rescue a person who has fallen through
the ice is to assume the prone position and reach out to her
with a stick. Keep your feet anchored on the shore so that you
aren't pulled into the water.

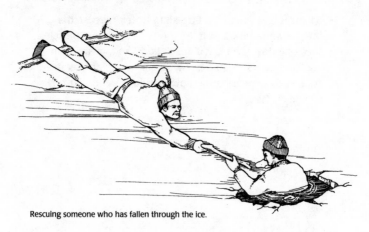

Rescuing someone who has fallen through the ice.

HYPOTHERMIA AND FROSTBITE

FROSTBITE

Frostbite is tissue injury or death caused by exposure to subfreezing cold. Here's how frostbite happens. When you become even mildly hypothermic, the blood vessels in your skin and extremities constrict in order to minimize further heat loss. The skin and subcutaneous tissues of your finger, toes, and other exposed parts freeze. Chilled arterioles just beneath the frozen tissues reflexively constrict, the blood in the capillaries becomes more viscous, and the flow of blood through these capillaries slows nearly to a halt. The blood becomes thick and syrupy, and clots form, blocking the capillary bed and depriving the tissues of badly needed oxygen and nutrients. Shunts running from arterioles to venules then divert blood away from the capillary beds. These shunts open and close in cycles, like the valves on a steam pipe, allowing waves of warm blood to surge into the feet from time to time. When your core temperature drops further, these shunts stay open for good and the tissues begin to freeze.

As the tissues cool, ice crystals form in the spaces outside the cells. These crystals then pull water out of the cells, dehydrating them, disrupting their cell membranes, and throwing a monkey wrench into their metabolic machinery.

PREDISPOSING FACTORS

Predisposing factors for frostbite include the following.

- *Ambient temperature.* Frostbite is more likely to occur in temperatures below 20°F (−6.7°C).

- *Windchill.* Wind accelerates the cooling process by increasing convective cooling.

- *High altitude.* It's colder in the mountains, the thinner air also seems to aggravate cold injury, and the storms are more violent.

- *Alcohol and drugs.* You won't know enough to come in out of the cold, or pull on a hat and mittens, if you're sloshed. You're also more likely to fall and break an arm or leg, increasing your risk of hypothermia *and* frostbite.

- *Conduction injury.* Metal and most other materials are much better heat conductors than air. On a cold day, a sled runner or the metal edge on a mountaineering ski extracts heat from your hand the way a magnet attracts iron filings. So does water.

- *Fatigue.* Vince Lombardi said, "Fatigue makes cowards of us all." It also makes us candidates for hypothermia and frostbite by depleting our energy reserves.

- *Underlying illness.* Diabetes and circulatory disorders impair the circulation to the extremities, setting the stage for frostbite.

- *Tobacco.* Nicotine puts the vise grip on the small arteries in the skin and extremities, opening the door for cold injury.

- *Previous frostbite.* Once you've been initiated into the Frostbite Club, you're a lifetime member and always vulnerable to repeat cold injury.

- *Deep snow.* Standing or walking in deep, loose snow is a recipe for frostbite. It is much colder deep down in the snow than on the surface.

SIGNS AND SYMPTOMS

Because of their distance from the warm core and because of their large surface-to-volume ratio, which predisposes to more rapid cooling, the feet, hands, ears, and nose are most vulnerable to frostbite.

The first response to cold is usually a stinging pain, followed by numbness and blanching of the tissue. This is *frostnip*. It looks like a small white patch on the cheeks, nose, or ears. Frostnip is easily treated by immediate rewarming.

Frostnip that is ignored progresses to *superficial frostbite*. This involves frozen skin and subcutaneous tissues. The skin remains bloodless, pale or gray, and cold to the touch. The tissue beneath the surface remains soft and pliable. A day or so after the injury, large blisters pop up like mushrooms. After a few days, the blisters heal, and a hard, dry *eschar* forms. This is a thick, black scar that separates from the underlying tissue in a few weeks and is replaced by new, red skin, which eventually takes on a normal appearance.

Deep frostbite involves freezing of superficial as well as deep structures, including nerve, muscle, tendon, and even bone. The affected part is purple or red, cool to the touch, and anesthetic. The limb is as hard as a piece of wood. In contrast to superficial frostbite, in which the injured part is sensitive, warm, and pink after rewarming, the part remains cold and blue after thawing. Small blood blisters may form after one to three weeks, and the part may remain swollen for months after. Eventually it will mummify and fall off.

TREATMENT

You can treat frostnipped hands anywhere, anytime, by breathing through cupped hands or by putting your hands in your armpits. But there's a time and a place for the treatment of frostbite. The place is *indoors*, and the time is when there is no chance that the thawed part will refreeze. *Avoid the freeze-thaw-refreeze cycle at all costs.* It is infinitely better to walk out of the wilderness on frostbitten feet than to thaw them out and risk the chance of their refreezing later. Before you start out for the warming hut, remove and replace all wet clothing and tight boots. And stay away from campfires en route.

Start thawing the injured part as soon as you get to a secure shelter. The key to recovery from frostbite is *rapid rewarming*. Fill a large container with 104° to 108°F (40°–42.2°C) water, and immerse the part in it. Remove all jewelry and constrictive clothing, and don't allow the part to rest on the bottom or sides of the vessel.

That frozen foot or hand will quickly cool the bath, so you'll have to add warm water at frequent intervals. Insure against scalding insensitive tissues by never using water warmer than an uninjured hand can tolerate and by thoroughly stirring the water before reimmersing the limb.

Rewarm until the skin becomes soft and flushed. And don't forget to warm the whole person! There is no point in rewarming a frozen foot if the circulation to the foot is still shut down due to hypothermia.

When you are done rewarming the limb, gently dry it with a clean towel; then elevate it on a pillow and fashion a protective cradle to keep blankets off it. Place sterile gauze or cotton between the digits to absorb moisture, and apply aloe vera or triple antibiotic ointment to the damaged skin.

Bathe the frostbitten part in a warm bath with mild soap twice a day. This cleans debris from the wounds, reduces the chance of infection, and stimulates circulation. It's also a good time to do gentle, active range-of-motion exercises to prevent stiffness in the digits. Don't disturb the blisters.

One or two aspirin or ibuprofen tablets twice a day may improve microcirculation and enhance healing. A few extra glasses of water or fruit juice each day will aid in rehydrating the frostbite/hypothermia victim and give the circulation a boost.

PREVENTION

A few words to the wise:

- Eat mountains of nutritious food in cold weather to keep that metabolic furnace stoked. (You'll get more bang for the buck from fats at low altitude.)

- Don't set out on a long trek too early in the morning or when the weather threatens to turn nasty.

- Tight boots have caused more cases of frostbite than the arctic express. Shun constrictive clothing, plastic boots, and tight crampon straps.

- Dress for success. Keep your head, neck, and face covered. On extremely cold days, tie a cloth over your face below your eyes and let it hang loosely. It will allow you to breathe and yet keep your face warm. Wear mittens instead of gloves, and keep them attached to a string draped around your neck. Keep your socks dry and wrinkle-free. Always bring along extra socks and mittens. You can stick a few feathers or some dry grass or moss inside your shoes for extra insulation.

- Wash your hands, face, and feet sparingly in cold weather. Soap and water remove protective oils; shaving removes the layer of dead cells that protects against the wind and cold. You want skin like a shark's in rough weather.

- Never touch metal with your bare hands in cold weather. Metal parts that must be touched with the bare hands should be wrapped with adhesive tape.

- Keep your fingernails and toenails trimmed.

- Allow several hours to recover from mild hypothermia.

- Avoid alcohol and tobacco.

- No matter what happens out there, don't panic. Remember, sweat accelerates evaporation and heat loss.

Sunburn and Heat Illness

SUNBURN

Sunburn pain and redness peak in 24 to 36 hours and resolve in two to three days. As soon as you realize that you have been burned, take a couple of aspirin or ibuprofen tablets and two more every four to six hours. Aspirin, ibuprofen, and naproxen are nonsteroidal anti-inflammatory drugs (NSAIDs), which block prostaglandins and will reduce the redness and pain. Cool compresses with milk and water or Burow's solution, or just lying in a cool stream, can provide merciful, if temporary, relief from the pain of sunburn. Soothing mentholated lotions and creams help too.

Symptom Chart: Sunburn and Heat Illness

Has victim been active in hot weather producing profuse sweating that then stops, leaving skin hot and dry to touch; body temperature rises?	**YES**	Evaluate and treat for heat stroke, pp. 88–89
NO		
Has victim been active in hot weather producing profuse sweating; skin is cold and clammy to touch?	**YES**	Evaluate and treat for heat exhaustion, p. 88
NO		
Has victim been active in hot weather producing profuse sweating with cramps in abdomen, legs, and/or arms?	**YES**	Evaluate and treat for heat cramps, p. 87
NO		
Is exposed skin hot, red, and painful?	**YES**	Evaluate and treat for sunburn, p. 86
NO		
Is there swelling of hands and/or feet on hot day?	**YES**	See heat edema, p. 87

HEAT ILLNESS

HANDLING THE HEAT

The body combats heat stress in two ways. Sweating is the first line of defense. Humans can withstand extreme heat and humidity as long as the sweating mechanism is intact and the salt and water lost in sweat are replenished. Heat is lost as sweat evaporates from the skin surface. As the body acclimatizes to heat and humidity, it develops the ability to produce sweat with a lower concentration of sodium chloride. The acclimatized individual also can produce a greater quantity of sweat. Acclimatization generally takes four to seven days.

The body's other major defense mechanism against heat stress is the dilatation of blood vessels in the skin. This allows for greater dissipation of heat through convection, radiation, and conduction.

TYPES

Heat cramps: Most people who develop heat cramps are in good physical condition but get into trouble when they engage in vigorous exercise or hard physical work on an unseasonably hot day. Their bodies can't handle the extra heat their muscles generate under such conditions. As a result, they sweat profusely and lose a large amount of salt (sodium chloride) in their sweat. The decreased sodium concentration in the blood causes their muscles to become more contractile, to the point where they go into spasm and cramp up. Unlike heat stroke victims, they sweat normally and their body temperatures do not rise.

Heat edema: Hormonal fluctuations and dilation of the blood vessels in the extremities and skin cause an expansion of the blood volume, which leads to *edema* (swelling) of the hands, feet, ankles, and legs. This is typically seen in unacclimated persons and the elderly. No treatment is needed.

Heat exhaustion: Heat exhaustion (heat prostration, heat collapse) is the most common form of heat illness. It typically afflicts unacclimated people who exercise hard during periods of high temperature and humidity (temperatures over 90°F, or 32.2°C; relative humidity over 60 percent), sweat profusely, and do not replace their water and electrolytes losses. But it also can strike sedentary individuals who sweat "insensibly" while sitting in the hot sun on a breezy day.

Heat exhaustion usually develops over a period of days. Headache, confusion, drowsiness, or euphoria are the usual harbingers, followed by a variety of symptoms that may include weakness, dizziness, nausea, vomiting, sweating, muscle cramps, chills, "goose bumps," and loss of coordination. The victim may collapse, and his skin is cold, clammy, and ashen gray. His temperature may be normal or up to 104°F (40°C). He'll recover in a few hours if you have him lie down in a cool spot and give him cold water to drink.

Heat stroke: Classic heat stroke is what kills the elderly and the chronically ill during a big-city heat wave. The victim sweats profusely at first, but her heat-dissipating mechanisms become so overwhelmed that she may experience headache, confusion, or drowsiness and then start to convulse or lapse into coma. Her body temperature soars, and once it exceeds 106°F (41.1°C), the blood and internal organs, especially the brain, heart, kidneys, and liver, start to bake.

Exertional heat stroke afflicts endurance athletes and others engaged in strenuous physical exercise in hot weather. The victim's pulse will be very rapid and his blood pressure low. Lung congestion, hyperventilation, vomiting, and diarrhea are common symptoms. The brain, which is exquisitely sensitive to heat, becomes swollen and congested when body temperature climbs during extreme conditions of heat and exercise. The victim may become agitated or delirious, lose muscle tone and control, and hallucinate or have a seizure before losing consciousness.

Treatment: Only heroic methods can prevent death. Keeping the ABCDEs in mind (see pages 12–14), stabilize the victim as well as you can, taking special care to protect her airway if she is unconscious. Then cool her as rapidly as possible. Remove her clothing and place her in ice bath or a lake or stream. After her temperature has been lowered to 102°F (38.9°C), place her in a cool, well-ventilated place and massage her skin. This stimulates the flow of cool blood from the skin to the overheated internal organs, and the return of warm blood from these organs to the skin, where its heat is dissipated. As soon as she is alert, give her cold fluids by mouth. Then arrange for medical evacuation.

PREVENTION

Here's how to stay cool when the going gets hot.

- Take a few days to become acclimatized to a hot climate before embarking on an arduous hike or climb.

- Stay hydrated. You can easily lose a liter or two of sweat an hour while hiking in a hot, humid environment, and you will lose even more after you acclimate. Furthermore, studies have shown that people never voluntarily drink as much water as they lose, and they usually replace only two-thirds of their net water losses. You cannot rely on thirst as a guide to replacing fluid losses on a hot day. If you haven't made a conscious effort to drink more water than you wanted, consider yourself to be dehydrated. To prevent dehydration, you should drink 8 ounces of water before exercise and 8 to 12 ounces (237–355 mL) every 20 to 30 minutes during exercise. The electrolytes lost in sweat are generally adequately replaced with meals or snacks. Let your urine be your guide to your level of hydration. If you are voiding good amounts of clear urine at regular intervals, you are replacing your fluid losses adequately. If you are producing scant, dark urine, you are dehydrated and need to drink more water.

- Wear absorbent, light-colored, loose-fitting clothing. Light colors absorb less light, and flowing clothing allows maximal evaporative heat loss.

- Take frequent dips in cold water streams or lakes.

- Accelerate evaporative heat loss after exercising in hot weather by dipping your clothes in water.

- Remain in a cool environment as much as possible, and avoid the midday sun.

Lightning Injuries

LIGHTNING'S PHYSICAL EFFECTS

Lightning can strike you in any of several ways. If you are caught out in the open during a lightning storm, you may be the victim of a *direct strike*. Wearing or carrying a metal object above shoulder level, such as a backpack or an ice axe, makes you an inviting target for a lightning strike. A *contact injury* occurs when you're holding a tent pole or some other object that is struck by lightning. A *splash injury* (also called *side flash* or *spray current*) classically occurs when lightning, seeking the path of least resistance, jumps from a tree to a person seeking refuge near the tree. Or it may jump from person to person in a group. Lightning striking the earth or a body of water causes an electric current to spread outward from the point of impact in concentric waves. This *ground current* (step voltage, stride voltage) can strike groups of hikers or swimmers. You also can be seriously injured by the *blast effect* of exploding or imploding air as lightning passes through it.

FLASHOVER EFFECT

A typical lightning bolt packs more punch than a cruise missile: 30 million volts and 250,000 amps of electrical energy. You'd think anyone struck by lightning would be turned into charcoal. But they aren't, thanks to the *flashover effect*. Lightning contact with the body is so brief (a millisecond or less) that there usually is not enough time for it to burn an entrance hole in the skin and pass internally. Instead, the current flashes over the outside of the body, vaporizing sweat and blasting off clothing and shoes. (Household current, on the other hand, causes the victim to "freeze" to the circuit. The skin is broken down and electricity surges through the tissues, baking internal organs.)

Symptom Chart: Lightning Injuries

Is victim unconscious after lightning strike? **YES**	Does victim have detectable pulse or breathing? **YES**	Does victim have pulse but is not breathing? **YES**	Clear airway, pp. 12–13, and perform rescue breathing, p. 13
NO	**NO**		
	Administer CPR, pp.17–18		
Does victim have feather or leaflike burns on skin or burns near metal objects such as jewelry? **YES**	Evaluate and treat for partial-thickness burns, pp. 31–32		
NO			
Does victim have injury to eye(s) after lightning strike? **YES**	See symptom chart for eye injuries, p. 67		
NO			
Is there hearing loss or bleeding from ears after lightning strike? **YES**	Evaluate and treat for ruptured eardrum, pp. 70–71		
NO			
Does victim complain of paralysis or partial paralysis after lightning strike? **YES**	Evaluate and treat for paralysis, pp. 51–52		

Lightning strike may blow your socks off yet cause amazingly minor injuries, such as transient blindness and deafness, confusion, muscle pain, and concussion. A heavier jolt might knock you out, crack a few bones, and paralyze your limbs. Or it might "strike you dead."

SIGNS AND SYMPTOMS OF LIGHTNING STRIKE

Cardiopulmonary: Lightning acts like a massive cosmic countershock, triggering a prolonged contraction of the heart muscle, followed by brief cardiac standstill. It also paralyzes the breathing center in the brain. Death is not instantaneous, though. The heart almost always resumes beating soon after the shock. But the brain takes longer to recover, and after going without oxygen for a few minutes, the heart goes into ventricular fibrillation. The victim dies of this *secondary cardiac arrest* unless a rescuer gives him mouth-to-mouth ventilation.

Central nervous system: A lightning strike to the head is like a Muhammad Ali punch—with brass knuckles. It can fracture your skull and scramble your brains, leaving you confused and amnesic for days. It can cause intracranial bleeding (see page 54). It may knock you out; leave you stunned, confused, and amnesic; and even change your personality. Two out of three lightning victims have transient paralysis of the legs, and one-third have paralyzed arms. Not surprisingly, lightning victims often develop a phobia of storms.

Burns: Flashover protects the skin from deep burns, but you may be scorched by belt buckles, jewelry, coins, or keys superheated by the lightning. Or the lightning may leave its calling card in the form of *feathering burns*, leaflike patterns where the skin has been imprinted by electron showers.

Circulation: Spasm of the blood vessels can cause the limbs to turn blue, mottled, and cold. Pulses in the arms and legs may be diminished.

Ears: The intense noise of thunder, which at ground zero approximates the sound of a battleship falling off a 50-story building, can cause temporary deafness. The shock wave or skull fracture may rupture your eardrums and cause vertigo and impaired balance.

Eyes: Lightning can cause a wide range of eye injuries, including transient or permanent blindness, corneal injuries, retinal detachment, bleeding into the front or back chamber of the eye, double vision, degeneration of the optic nerves, and loss of color vision. Cataracts are common and usually develop within a few days of injury. Lightning also can cause the pupils to become widely dilated and unresponsive to light. Fixed, dilated pupils are not a sign of death in a lightning victim.

Blast effect: The explosive force of lightning may rupture the liver, spleen or kidneys or blow you off a mountain ledge, resulting in fractured ribs, skull, limbs, spine, or pelvis.

TREATMENT OF LIGHTNING INJURIES

RECOGNIZING LIGHTNING INJURY

Lightning strikes in the blink of an eye, and if you aren't on the scene when it happens, you may be unsure of whether you are dealing with the victim of a seizure, stroke, heart attack, drug overdose, or foul play. If you come across a person lying unconscious on the trail with her clothes in shreds and bruises all over her body, you might logically conclude that she's been assaulted. But if she is unconscious or dazed, has burns in a feather or leaflike pattern on her skin and blood draining from her ears, and her arms and legs are cold, blue, and mottled, you can safely assume that she's been struck by lightning.

FIRST RESPONSE

Remember the ABCDEs: *a*irway, *b*reathing, *c*irculation, *d*isability, and *e*xpose (see pages 12–14). If the victim isn't breathing and has no pulse, start CPR. If you are successful in restoring a heart beat, continue breathing for the victim until she starts breathing on her own. Then do a systematic search for other injuries, making sure that you keep her neck and back immobilized if you have reason to suspect spinal injury. Splint any fractures, attend to any wounds or burns, and treat her for hypothermia if she's been exposed to the elements for any length of time.

GROUP THERAPY

Mass casualties are traditionally *triaged* (sorted) into three groups.

1. those victims who are going to survive no matter what is done for them

2. those who are going to die no matter what is done for them

3. those who are going to die if something isn't done for them *right now*

The first two groups are ignored until those in the last group are stabilized. But the rules change when you're dealing with a group of people who have been struck by lightning. Now you "resuscitate the dead." People who are moaning and groaning are going to make it. Those in cardiac arrest have a good chance for survival if they are given CPR, particularly if you get to them before the heart goes into secondary arrest due to lack of oxygen. (Remember, if you are able to restore a heartbeat, prolonged artificial breathing may be necessary.)

When the third group has been attended to, then go back to the ABCDEs as you evaluate and treat the other victims and prepare them for evacuation. Wounds, fractures and dislocations, burns, head injuries, and chest and abdominal injuries are treated in the usual way. Ruptured eardrums don't require immediate treatment but will need eventual medical evaluation, as will many eye injuries (see pages 66–68). Cold, blue extremities are often a sign of shock or hypothermia but in this setting are more likely due to vascular spasm and should regain their normal color and temperature within a few hours. Naturally, if there are other signs of shock, treat the patient for shock. Paralysis after lightning strike normally resolves within a few hours also. If it doesn't, you'll have to assume that the victim has a brain or spinal cord injury and arrange for medical evacuation.

LIGHTNING INJURY PREVENTION

WHAT YOU SHOULD DO IN A LIGHTNING STORM

Lightning is one of nature's great spectacles, but you don't want to become part of the show. Here's how to stay out of trouble during a thunderstorm.

- Seek refuge in a building or an all-metal vehicle.

- If you see St. Elmo's fire on nearby objects (or yourself) or feel your hair standing on end, hit the deck.

- Stay out of tents (tent poles can be lightning rods).

- Put down tent poles or other metal objects, remove metal objects from your hair, and take off hobnailed boots.

- If you are in a forest, wait out the storm in a low area under a thick growth of small trees.

- If you are in the open, stay away from single trees, corn stalks, and hay stacks. Find a dry cave or a ditch, and crouch down with your feet close together. Or lie curled up on the ground on a rubber or plastic raincoat.

- If you are with a group of people, spread out to avoid ground current and splashes. Also stay out of the water. Groups of people in the water have been killed by ground current.

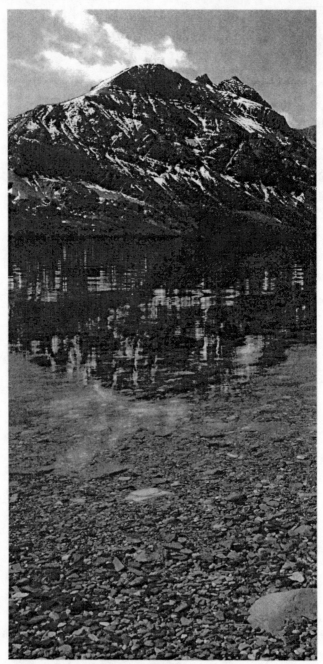

Lake McDonald, Glacier National Park, Montana

LIGHTNING MYTHS AND SUPERSTITIONS

- *"The safest place to wait out a lightning storm outdoors is under a tree."* Only if you're in the mood for a little excitement. Lightning tends to strike the highest object in an area. If the tree you're standing under is hit by lightning, you're going to get zapped too.

- *"You'll always be safe from lightning in a car."* Only if it's a hardtop. All-metal cars deflect the charge around the metal skin and down into the ground. Open-frame vehicles and convertibles won't protect you from lightning.

- *"Lightning never strikes on a clear day."* Lightning can strike during a snowstorm, a sandstorm, a volcanic eruption, or seemingly out of the blue when a long horizontal flash turns earthward miles from the cloud that spawned it.

- *"Lightning strike is usually fatal."* Wrong. Lightning kills only about 30 percent of its victims, and timely CPR would save most of those.

- *"If you hear thunder, you're safe from lightning strike."* Well, for a while, anyway, since thunder precedes lightning by several seconds. But you won't hear the one that hits you.

- *"It's dangerous to touch a lightning strike victim."* No. The electric current passes through the victim's body in a fraction of a second and is gone.

- *"Lightning injuries are no different from other electrical injuries."* Lightning usually passes outside the body, so injuries are usually less severe than those caused by generated electricity, which traverses the body and damages internal organs.

- *"Lightning victims are in a state of suspended animation and may be revived after prolonged resuscitation."* Lightning confers no protective effect on brain metabolism. Breathing and heartbeat have to be restored within minutes to allow any chance for survival in a person who has been "struck dead."

- *"Lightning never strikes twice."* Ask the owner of the Empire State Building. It's hit by lightning thousands of times a year. So are many mountain peaks and radio and television antennas. Whatever it is that attracts lightning to an object will attract it repeatedly.

Drowning and Near-Drowning

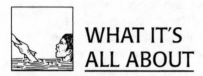

WHAT IT'S ALL ABOUT

DEFINITIONS

Let's define a few terms before we get in over our heads. *Immersion* is the state of being in the water with your head out. *Submersion* is the state of being under the water, head and all. *Aspiration* is the inhalation of water or stomach contents into the lungs. *Drowning* is death by asphyxia following submersion. *Near-drowning* is at least temporary survival after being submersed.

HOW IT HAPPENS

Here's what happens when you drown.

1. First you panic. You kick, scream, and thrash about like a wild man or woman.

2. All that to-do makes you too tired to keep your head above water, so you start holding your breath. (You also swallow lots of water, which distends your stomach and makes you vomit.)

3. When you can hold your breath no longer, you start gasping for air and inhale enough water to block your airway. This leads to a severe drop in blood oxygen content, and you pass out, aspirate more water, and suffocate if you're not pulled from the water and resuscitated in time. When the brain goes without oxygen for more than four or five minutes, it's damaged irreversibly, and when the heart is deprived of oxygen for that length of time, it fibrillates.

Symptom Chart: Drowning and Near-Drowning

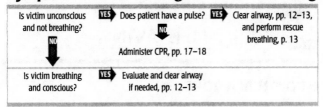

Is victim unconscious and not breathing? **YES** → Does patient have a pulse? **YES** → Clear airway, pp. 12–13, and perform rescue breathing, p. 13

NO → Administer CPR, pp. 17–18

Is victim unconscious and not breathing? ↓ **NO**

Is victim breathing and conscious? **YES** → Evaluate and clear airway if needed, pp. 12–13

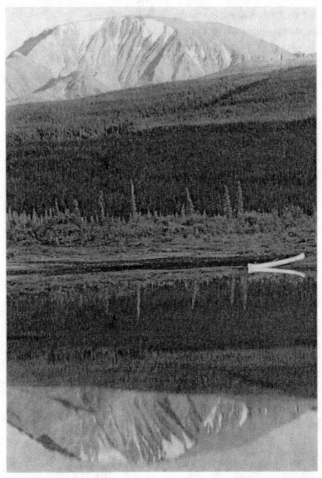

The Yukon, Canada

BASIC LIFESAVING

THROW HIM A ROPE

The first rule for any would-be rescuer is to not become a victim yourself. Panic can endow the drowning person with the power of Sampson. If you jump in the water and swim right out to him, he is liable to crawl right on top of you.

The safest approach to the person in distress in the water is to extend a long stick or pole out to him. Let him grab the end of the stick and pull himself in. If a rope is handy, throw it to him and pull him in.

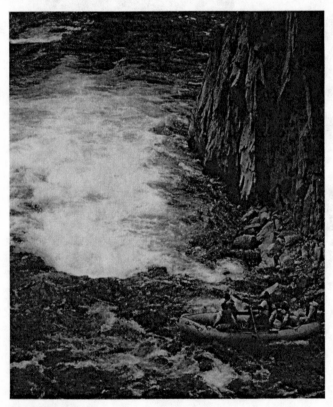

Salmon River, Idaho

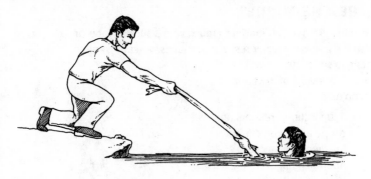

Rescuing the near-drowning victim from the shore.

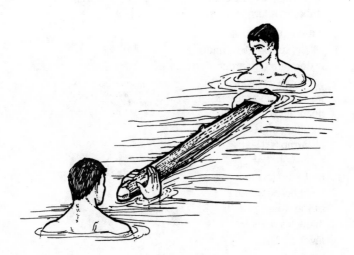

Rescuing the near-drowning victim with a branch or log.

RESCUE CARRIES

If the victim is too far out to reach with a stick or rope, and you are trained in water rescue techniques, you are going to have to swim out and get him. Here is a review of the basic techniques.

1. If the victim is rational and cooperative, you can use the *tired swimmer's carry*. Approach him from the front, and tell him to put his hands on your shoulders. Then use the breast stroke to return to shore.

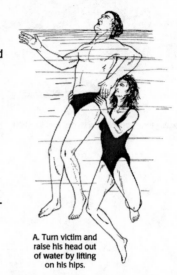

A. Turn victim and raise his head out of water by lifting on his hips.

2. If the victim is flailing wildly, swim to him underwater, turn him around so that he is facing away from you, and raise his head out of the water by lifting under his armpits. Next, place your hand under his jaw to keep his head out of the water, and allow his body to level off. Then reach your arm around his chest and sidestroke to shore. If he panics, join your hands and just keep his face out of the water until he calms down. Or escape by letting go of him and sinking down into the water.

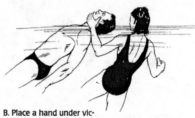

B. Place a hand under victim's jaw to keep his head out of water and allow his body to level off.

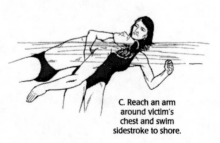

C. Reach an arm around victim's chest and swim sidestroke to shore.

The cross-chest carry.

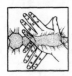

TREATMENT

CPR

If the victim is in cardiac arrest, start CPR as soon as you get him on shore (see pages 17–18). If the airway is blocked, perform the Heimlich maneuver (see pages 19–20) or remove mud and debris manually. Continue CPR until you revive the victim or emergency medical personnel take over. If you're in the wilderness, continue CPR until the victim has warmed to ambient temperature. Remember, the cold-water drowning victim is not dead until he's warm and dead.

POSTIMMERSION SYNDROME

Some near-drowning victims appear to be fine after they are pulled out of the water but develop severe shortness of breath minutes to hours after the incident. This is called *secondary drowning* or the *postimmersion syndrome*. Anyone who has been submersed for more than a minute or two should be evaluated medically and observed for the development of post-immersion syndrome.

Spider, Scorpion, Insect, and Snake Bites and Stings

 ## <u>SPIDER FACTS</u>

Spiders are *arachnids*, a class that includes scorpions, ticks, and mites. They live everywhere and are prodigious travelers, the hobos of the arachnid world. Up to 2 million may live in an acre of grassland and 265,000 in an acre of woodland.

Spiders have two major body segments (the cephalothorax and the abdomen), eight legs, a pair of feelers, and a pair of jaws. At the end of each jaw is a hollow fang, which connects to a venom sac in the cephalothorax. Spider venom contains potent chemicals that paralyze and partially digest prey.

Spiders are meat eaters, dining mostly on other insects. The larger ones also feast on frogs, lizards, and fish. Most spiders are harmless to humans, but about a dozen of the thousands of species that make their homes in the United States can cause at least mild illness. The bites of some can be fatal.

BLACK WIDOW SPIDERS

Latrodectus mactans, the black widow, is found in every state but Alaska. The female is the size of a thumbnail and has a shiny, coal black body; a prominent, spherical

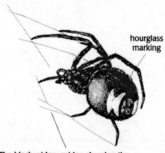

hourglass marking

The black widow spider, showing the characteristic hourglass marking.

Symptom Chart: Spider, Scorpion, Insect, and Snake Bites and Stings

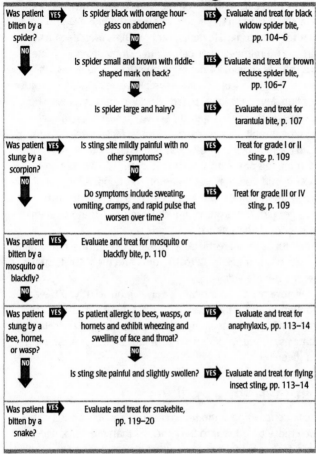

Was patient bitten by a spider? **YES**	Is spider black with orange hourglass on abdomen? **YES**	Evaluate and treat for black widow spider bite, pp. 104–6
NO	**NO**	
	Is spider small and brown with fiddle-shaped mark on back? **YES**	Evaluate and treat for brown recluse spider bite, pp. 106–7
	NO	
	Is spider large and hairy? **YES**	Evaluate and treat for tarantula bite, p. 107
Was patient stung by a scorpion? **YES**	Is sting site mildly painful with no other symptoms? **YES**	Treat for grade I or II sting, p. 109
NO	**NO**	
	Do symptoms include sweating, vomiting, cramps, and rapid pulse that worsen over time? **YES**	Treat for grade III or IV sting, p. 109
Was patient bitten by a mosquito or blackfly? **YES**	Evaluate and treat for mosquito or blackfly bite, p. 110	
NO		
Was patient stung by a bee, hornet, or wasp? **YES**	Is patient allergic to bees, wasps, or hornets and exhibit wheezing and swelling of face and throat? **YES**	Evaluate and treat for anaphylaxis, pp. 113–14
NO	**NO**	
	Is sting site painful and slightly swollen? **YES**	Evaluate and treat for flying insect sting, pp. 113–14
Was patient bitten by a snake? **YES**	Evaluate and treat for snakebite, pp. 119–20	

stomach; and a characteristic red or orange hourglass marking on her undersurface. The male is half the size of the female, too small to have a harmful bite.

After mating with and then eating her husband, the female finds a dark corner, weaves a coarse web, and suspends her eggs in it. Although generally regarded as timid, the female black widow fiercely defends her eggs. She can be downright nasty, and her venom, a neurotoxin that causes sustained muscle spasms, is more potent than that of a cobra or a coral snake. Happily, she doesn't inject much of it into her human victims.

Bite signs and symptoms: The black widow spider bite can produce a sharp sting or it may be painless; many victims don't even realize that they have been bitten. They may notice a small bump and some redness at the bite site and have no other symptoms. However, other victims aren't so lucky. Thirty to 60 minutes after being bitten, they develop tremendous muscle spasms of the large muscles of the limbs, abdomen, and lower back. Other symptoms may include profuse sweating, fever, elevated blood pressure, thready pulse, shortness of breath, slurred speech, excessive salivation, muscle twitching, vomiting, weakness, seizures, facial swelling, droopy eyelids, and *priapism* (prolonged penile erection). If you're bitten in the leg or genitals, your abdomen will become rigid as a board, and you may get taken off to the operating room for an operation you don't need. If you're bitten on the arm, you'll get terrific spasms of the chest muscles that can mimic the pain of a heart attack.

Painful as they are, black widow spider bites are rarely fatal. The symptoms peak in 12 to 18 hours and then slowly subside over the next few days.

Treatment: Clean the bite wound, apply ice if you have it, and then head for the nearest hospital. Treatment there will consist of blood pressure monitoring, intravenous narcotics or sedatives for muscle spasms and, if indicated, administration of antivenin.

BROWN SPIDERS

Loxosceles spiders, the brown recluse and its cousins, are much more of a threat to backpackers than are black widows. There are more of them, both sexes bite, and their bites can cause *necrotic arachnidism*: gangrenous ulcers, systemic poisoning, and even death. The brown recluse is a medium-sized, fawn to dark brown spider. It's known as the "fiddle-back" spider because of the violin-shaped figure on its back. It ranges throughout the United States but prefers hot, arid environments. True to its name, it remains secluded during the day, venturing out at night to hunt.

Bite signs and symptoms: The bite of the brown spider may be virtually painless. More commonly, it causes a sharp, stinging pain that gives way after a few hours to aching and itching as chemicals in the venom constrict the blood vessels in the area of the bite, shutting off blood flow to the skin and underlying fat. The skin around the bite swells, and large, violet blisters develop. These blisters become progressively darker and evolve into a thick black scab, which sloughs off after a few weeks, leaving a deep ulcer. Severe bites can be associated with fever, joint pains, rash, weakness, nausea and vomiting, *hemolytic anemia* (destruction of red blood cells), kidney failure, and even death.

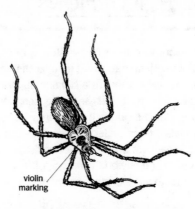

violin marking

The brown recluse spider, showing the characteristic violin marking.

Treatment: If the bite is mild, apply cold packs to the bite and elevate and immobilize the bitten extremity. Severe bites require hospital treatment.

TARANTULAS

Bird spiders, funnel-web spiders, and trapdoor spiders are *tarantulas*, big, furry spiders that live long and move slowly. About forty species of tarantulas are native to the United States. Their bites resemble bee stings and require nothing more than elevation, immobilization, and a mild analgesic.

SCORPIONS

Scorpions look like small lobsters with an elongated abdominal segment that curves up over the body and ends in a *telson*. The telson contains a stinging apparatus that scorpions use to kill insects, spiders, and other scorpions when they go foraging at night. During the day, they burrow in the sand or hide in fallen trees, under rocks and logs, in piles of wood or brush, or beneath houses and outbuildings. Scorpions have poor vision and rely on their sense of feel, stinging any moving object that touches or steps on them.

SIGNS AND SYMPTOMS OF SCORPION STING

Nonlethal scorpions rarely cause more than a mild sting and a little redness at the sting site. *Centuroides exilicauda*, the "bark scorpion," is the only scorpion native to the United States that causes severe toxicity. It is yellow to brown in color, up to 2 inches (5 cm) long, has a knob at the base of its stinger, and may have dark stripes down its back. It lives in desert areas of the Southwestern United States and in northern Mexico. *Centruroides*'s venom causes prolonged hyperstimulation of the nervous system, resulting in four grades of *envenomation* (poisoning).

1. local pain and/or tingling at sting site

2. as above, plus pain and/or tingling at other sites

3. cranial nerve dysfunction (slurred speech, difficulty swallowing, hypersalivation, blurred vision, abnormal eye movements) *or* neuromuscular dysfunction (restlessness, jerking of limbs, wild involuntary shaking of the limbs)

4. both cranial nerve and neuromuscular dysfunction

Most envenomations cause only mild pain for a few hours. In more severe envenomations, pain intensifies over a period of a few minutes to an hour and the area becomes exquisitely sensitive to the touch. Tapping the sting site sends pain and tingling sensations shooting up the arm or leg. The victim becomes jumpy and jittery and may experience hypertension, headache, hyperthermia, abdominal cramps, vomiting, rapid pulse, heavy sweating, wheezing, and respiratory distress.

TREATMENT AND PREVENTION

Treat grades 1 and 2 envenomations with cold packs, analgesics, and a watchful eye for signs of progression to a higher grade. If the victim has symptoms of grade 3 or 4 envenomation, take her to a hospital, where an antivenin may be administered.

To prevent scorpion stings, wear shoes when you walk outside at night, shake out your shoes and clothing each morning and your sleeping bags before turning in at night, and keep your hands out of potential scorpion hideouts, especially woodpiles and under rocks, logs, and tree bark.

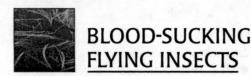

BLOOD-SUCKING FLYING INSECTS

MOSQUITOES

These winged vampires rely on an exquisite sense of smell to find a blood meal, and carbon dioxide on the skin or in the breath really perks up their taste buds. Some prefer to feed at night, others during the day, but most will bite at twilight. During the day, they rest in cool, dark places. They breed in tidal marshes and flooded lowlands near lakes and rivers, and they find some humans tastier than others, for reasons unknown.

The problem starts when a female mosquito, attracted by carbon dioxide and human sweat, alights on your skin and takes a meal. She drills her syringelike nose under the skin and injects saliva, which contains a blood-thinning substance, a few proteins, and possibly a few microorganisms, into the bite. The result is an itchy wheal; within 12 to 24 hours, the area becomes red, swollen, and more itchy.

Treatment: Apply ice to minimize the swelling and itching in the first few minutes after a mosquito bite. Calamine or antihistamine lotion will decrease redness and itching. More intense reactions may require diphenhydramine, 25 or 50 mg by mouth every six hours.

BLACKFLIES

These small (2 to 4 mm) humpbacked bloodsuckers breed in fast-flowing streams and take over the woods in many northern areas early in the summer. They are day feeders and rely mostly on visual cues to find a blood meal. The adults prefer open, sunny areas, but they are attracted to dark, moving objects. They hate dark *places*, such as the insides of tents and vehicles. They seem to have a fascination for eyes, ears, nostrils, and whatever is under your clothing. The bite—a large, bleeding puncture—becomes red, swollen, itchy, and painful, and it may take weeks for the weeping, crusted sores to heal.

Treatment: Treatment consists of local wound care.

HOW TO PROTECT YOURSELF AGAINST FLYING INSECTS

THE NUMBERS GAME

If you wipe out 99 percent of the mosquitoes circling around inside your tent on a summer night, you have won the battle but lost the war. One female mosquito can produce 20 million progeny in a single season. You can't lick mosquitoes, flies, and gnats with overwhelming force, but you can outsmart them by taking a three-pronged approach focusing on avoidance, physical barriers, and chemical deterrence.

AVOIDANCE

Follow these rules to avoid confrontations.

- Avoid tall grasses, bushes, animal burrows, hollow trees and logs, caves, and other mosquito hangouts during the day.
- Stay indoors at dusk.
- Stay out of the woods during the early part of the season.
- Use lights sparingly.
- Camp on high, dry, open ground, and keep a campfire going. The smoke will usually keep the mosquitoes away.

PHYSICAL BARRIERS

- Wear loose-fitting, brightly colored clothing (long pants and long-sleeved shirts with a T-shirt underneath) made of tightly woven fabric, and pad it with leaves, grass, or bark.
- Protect your head and neck with a brightly colored, full-brimmed hat.
- Use a head net when the bugs are really swarming. If you don't have one, tie off the arms and neck of your undershirt and slip it over your head. Keep if off your scalp by padding your head with bark or leaves, and cut slits for your eyes.

CHEMICAL DETERRENCE

You have two trump cards in your battle against mosquitoes, flies, and gnats: DEET and permethrin. DEET is the most effective repellent available. Use a product containing no more than 35 percent DEET, and apply it directly to all exposed skin but not near the eyes, mouth, nose, sunburned areas, cuts, or rashes. Reapply as needed, and wash it off when you no longer need it.

Permethrin is a safe, effective insecticide that adheres to clothing for months. It's available as a spray or a solution. Commercial products include Duranon Tick Repellent, Permanone Tick Repellent, Coulston's Permethrin Arthropod Repellent, and Expel. To spray clothing with permethrin, lay the garment out and spray it front and back until the fabric is damp; then hang it up to dry. For longer protection, use the soaking technique. First make up a solution: pour 2 ounces (59 mL) of permethrin into a waterproof bag, add 1½ cups (355 mL) of water, and shake twice. Then fold the garment lengthwise, roll it up, and tie the middle with a string. Place the garment in the bag, shake it twice, and let it soak for at least 2½ hours. Then remove it, untie the string, and hang it up until it dries.

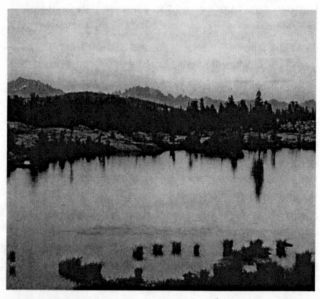

High Sierra, California

  SPIDER, SCORPION, INSECT, AND SNAKE BITES AND STINGS

STINGING INSECTS

STING OPERATION

The average bee weighs about as much as a candle flame but packs the firepower of a miniature F-16. Instead of bomb racks, they have venom sacs attached to their stingers. The sting of a bee, wasp, hornet, yellow jacket, or ant (all members of the order Hymenoptera) means instant pain. It may also mean instant death if you are one of the many people who are allergic to bees.

Honeybees are kamikazes. Their barbed stingers and venom sacs remain embedded in the skin after stinging, and when they fly away, they are disemboweled and soon die.

If you disturb a nest, you're liable to be swarmed. The first bee on the scene releases *pheromones*, chemical signals that trigger aggressive behavior in other bees. One sting will cause pain, swelling, and redness. Multiple bee stings can cause massive swelling, vomiting and diarrhea, shortness of breath, shock, and collapse. Receiving 100 to 200 stings can be fatal.

Allergic reactions to bees range in severity from simple hives, nausea, and dizziness to *anaphylaxis*, a severe allergic reaction that causes swelling of the face, lips, and throat; wheezing; shock; and respiratory arrest. Most allergic reactions develop within a few minutes, although they may be delayed as long as six hours.

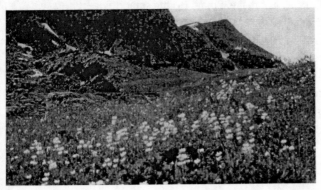

Rockies, Colorado

TREATMENT AND PREVENTION

First check to see if there is a stinger present and remove it if there is. Then take an aspirin tablet, moisten it, and tape it over the sting site. The pain will disappear almost immediately.

If you are allergic to bees, you'll need a shot of adrenaline and an antihistamine if you develop any sign of a severe reaction (wheezing, swelling of the face and throat, collapse). Kits are available (Ana-Kit, EpiPen) that have preloaded syringes of adrenaline and diphenhydramine tablets for emergencies. If you have had a severe bee sting reaction in the past, apply a light tourniquet just above the sting site if it's on an arm or leg.

Here are some strategies you can use to prevent unpleasant encounters with stinging insects.

- Don't leave food out in the open. Yellow jackets are attracted to meat, fruits, and fruit syrup.

- Take great pains to avoid hymenopteran nests, or you will *be* in great pain.

- Know where you're likely to encounter stinging insects. Honeybees favor rock crevices and hollow trees; you'll see wasp nests hanging from trees; yellow jackets usually nest underground in animal burrows and tree stumps; and fire ants are found throughout the southern United States in mound nests in open, grassy areas.

- Stay out of the way of bees or other hymenopterans flying in a straight line. They may be making a "beeline" to their nest and may become aggressive if they think you are blocking their way.

- If you have an encounter with a bee, don't slap at it. That will just make it mad. Do the smart thing—run. Take refuge in a tent, building, vehicle, or dark, shady area.

- Be especially wary of bees on cloudy days. Like most of us, they are more irritable when the sky is gray and it's threatening to rain.

- Keep your shoes on when walking in the woods.

- If you have a history of bee-sting allergy, take a bee-sting kit along with you into the wilderness.

SNAKES

IDENTIFYING SNAKES

Two families of venomous snakes are indigenous to the United States: the Elapidae, which includes the eastern and western coral snake, and the Crotalidae, or pit vipers, which includes copperheads, cottonmouths (water moccasins), and rattlesnakes.

Although the eastern coral snake is far deadlier, pit vipers have the country blanketed from coast to coast and are responsible for most of the snakebites reported in this country.

Snake anatomy: You've got to be able to "get a make" on the snake that bites you, since treatment depends on the perpetrator's species. Pit vipers have four distinguishing characteristics.

1. a heat-sensing *pit* between the eye and nostril on each side of the head (these pits can detect changes in temperature as slight as 0.007°F, or 0.003°C)

2. cat-like vertical, *elliptical pupils*

3. a *triangular head*, which is distinct from the rest of the body

4. a single row of *subcaudal* (under the tail) scales

Pit vipers also have heavy bodies and upper fangs that fold back when they aren't biting. Rattlesnakes have *rattles*, of course, which are thick, interlocking skin segments that accumulate as the snake sheds its skin from time to time. Pit vipers range in size from about 1½ feet (0.5 m), for a *pygmy rattlesnake*,

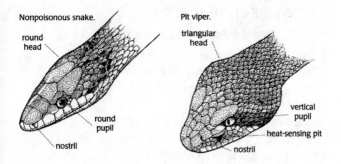

Nonpoisonous snake.

round head

round pupil

nostril

Pit viper.

triangular head

vertical pupil

heat-sensing pit

nostril

to over 8 feet (2.4 m), for *eastern and western diamondback rattlesnakes.*

Coral snakes are smaller (1 to 4 feet, or 0.3 to 1.2 m), skinnier snakes, with short, fixed fangs; alternating bands of red, black, yellow, or white bands encircling their bodies; black snouts; round pupils; and a double row of subcaudal scales.

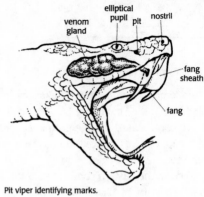

Pit viper identifying marks.

Coral snake.

SNAKE PHYSIOLOGY 101

Snakes have poor vision, but they are very sensitive to ground vibrations. Their keen sense of smell derives from their forked tongues, which they use to pick up scents.

Snakes are cold-blooded animals, so their body temperature fluctuates with the ambient temperature. But they prefer to stay in the 81° to 90°F (27°–32°C) range. So they sun themselves on rocks on cool days, feed at night during the warm season, and hibernate during the winter.

Snakes are most aggressive when they are emerging from or preparing for hibernation, so more bites occur in the early summer and early fall.

THE CAST OF CHARACTERS

Here's a rogues' gallery of venomous American snakes.

- *Cottonmouth (water moccasin).* A semiaquatic snake found in lakes and swamps in the Northeast and in lakes, ponds, lagoons, and bayous in the Southeast. Its mouth has a distinctive white lining.

- *Copperhead.* Inhabits meadows, mountains, and abandoned buildings in the Northeast, swamps and uplands in the southeast and central United States, and wooded hills

SPIDER, SCORPION, INSECT, AND SNAKE BITES AND STINGS

in central Texas. Usually docile, but never trust a snake who can climb trees.

- *Timber rattlesnake.* Prefers wooded and mountainous areas in the Northeast and wooded, rocky hills in the Southeast. Likes to sun itself on rocky ledges.

- *Pygmy rattlesnake.* Prefers swamps, marshes, lakes, and rivers in the Southeast and grasslands in southeastern Arizona, New Mexico, and southern Texas.

- *Eastern diamondback rattlesnake.* A big, mean snake who hangs out in low coastal areas, dry pine woods, and scrub palmetto. The biggest and most dangerous rattlesnake.

- *Eastern coral snake.* Found in grasslands, dry woods, and along streams in the southeastern states and Texas. Won't bite unless provoked, but then won't let go.

- *Western (Sonoran) coral snake.* A denizen of the Great Sonoran Desert of Arizona and New Mexico. Its potent venom can cause total paralysis.

- *Massasauga rattlesnake.* Inhabits prairies, dry wooded areas, woodpiles, grasslands, hayfields, and cellars in the central states, and prairies in Texas and Arizona. This is a reclusive snake that bites only if cornered.

- *Prairie rattlesnake.* Favors rock hills, grasslands, and open mountain slopes in the central states and grasslands and hills in the southwestern states.

- *Sidewinder.* They named a missile after this snake. Hangs out in sandy flats, dunes, and arid, rocky hillsides in southwestern and western deserts. Rests with its body buried in the sand.

- *Western diamondback rattlesnake.* Found in open and cultivated areas and near farm buildings in the Southwest and southwestern California. Aggressive, like its cousin, the eastern diamondback.

- *Northern Pacific rattlesnake.* Lives in semiarid areas to 11,000 feet (3,353 m) in northern California, Oregon, and Washington.

- *Southern Pacific rattlesnake.* Found in semiarid areas in southern California.

MODUS OPERANDI

Snakes don't hypnotize their prey, nor do they necessarily hiss or give a warning rattle before they attack. Nor do they have to be coiled to strike. They don't even have to be alive to strike. A primitive reflex enables a severed rattlesnake head to bite for 20 to 60 minutes after decapitation. A 17-year-old boy was envenomated when he impaled his wrist on the fangs of a dried snake head!

The potency of a snake's venom and the amount it injects depends on its age and size, the timing of its last meal (it takes three weeks to replenish the venom after a bite), time of year (venom is more concentrated when the snake emerges from hibernation in the spring), and the species. The eastern diamondback, for instance, can inject up to 800 mg of very potent venom, compared to the cottonmouth's 145 mg of moderately potent venom and the copperhead's 40 to 70 mg of mildly toxic venom. The eastern coral snake, on the other hand, only injects 2 to 6 mg of venom, but it is 30 times as potent by volume as most rattlesnakes' venom.

Rattlesnake venom is a witch's brew of enzymes that destroy muscle and fat, oxidize amino acids, trigger the release of histamine from cells, cause small blood vessels to leak, rupture red blood cells, and disrupt the normal blood clotting mechanism. But not everyone who is bitten develops an *envenomation syndrome*. Around 20 percent of bites are *dry bites* (no venom is injected), and in another 10 percent the snake injects an insignificant amount of venom. If you're not in that happy 30 percent, you've got problems, depending on

- *Your age and size.* Adults rarely die of snakebite, but children can have severe reactions. The bigger you are, the less vulnerable you are to snake poisoning.

- *Your health.* Snakebite is especially dangerous in old people, menstruating and pregnant women, and anyone with hypertension, peptic ulcers, diabetes, or bleeding disorders.

- *Location and depth of the bite.* Snakebites on the head, trunk, and arms are especially dangerous. Injection of venom directly into a blood vessel can put you right into shock.

- *Duration of the bite.* Rattlesnakes bite and run. Coral snakes don't know when to let go.

SIGNS AND SYMPTOMS OF SNAKEBITE

Rattlesnake bites don't hurt much at first. You'll feel a little burning sensation and see a fang mark or two, with a little bleeding. But then enzymes in the venom start to liquify your connective tissues, allowing the venom to spread through the tissues. Other enzymes ravage muscle fibers and fat, denature proteins, rupture cell walls, and lay waste to the tissues around the bite. Within hours, your arm or leg swells up like a balloon and turns blue and purple. Blebs and blisters pop out all around the bite site. By this time, the pain has become intense, you feel weak and nauseated, and you're sweating profusely. As the venom seeps into blood vessels, it ruptures red blood cells and disrupts the clotting system, causing widespread bleeding. By now, several hours after the bite, you're in shock.

Coral snake bites: Coral snake venom contains a neurotoxin similar to the curare that South American Indians used to dab their arrowheads in. The bite of the eastern coral snake is painless and produces little swelling and no blisters, discoloration, or necrosis. There may not even be any fang marks. All you feel is a little tingling and muscle twitching at the bite site. You may shrug it off, thinking the snake was nonvenomous. But the neurotoxin works its way through your bloodstream, attaches to your nerves, and starts to exert its grisly effects after a few hours. You may become euphoric and then get drowsy or nauseated. Later you find it hard to swallow, and you start drooling. Your vision becomes blurred, your eyelids droop, and then your arms and legs become weak and paralyzed. The gruesome process ends in asphyxiation. Fortunately, only 40 percent of coral snake bites cause serious envenomation, and fatalities are rare. Western coral snakes rarely bite humans and when they do cause only mild neurological symptoms.

TREATMENT OF SNAKEBITE

It's been said that the only thing you need to treat snakebite is car keys, so you can drive yourself to a hospital for proper treatment. Many of the traditional measures, such as tourniquets and incision and suctioning, are fraught with danger and of questionable value. Ice doesn't seem to influence the spread of venom in tissues, and you don't need frostbite on top of snakebite. Pressure wraps, although they may delay spread of the venom for a while, do not really prevent swelling, discoloration, and clotting abnormalities and bleeding.

These are the things that you *should* do after being bitten by a snake.

1. Move out of the snake's striking range (about the length of the snake).

2. Stay cool.

3. If you were bitten by a coral snake, apply a constricting band—but loosely, so that it barely indents the skin. A shoelace or strips of cloth will do the job.

4. Gently cleanse the wound, and apply a sterile dressing. Splint a bitten upper extremity, or simply place it in a sling and keep it at heart level or lower. Immobilizing the bitten part minimizes necrosis and delays spread of the venom into the bloodstream. The same logic dictates that you try not to move around too much.

5. Do *not* use pressure dressings, tourniquets, or cold packs or attempt to incise the tissue and suck out the venom. These techniques do not work.

6. Have your partners bring you to a hospital. You can walk to a car if it's less than a 20-minute walk. Otherwise, you should be carried out by litter, horse, or helicopter. If there's going to be a long wait for transportation, let the bitten extremity hang down in a dependent position. If you are alone, start walking. You probably will be able to walk for several hours before severe envenomation symptoms start.

7. Bring the snake with you (if it's dead) so that it can be identified at the hospital.

PREVENTION OF SNAKEBITE

Here are some tips on snakebite prevention.

1. Stay out of snake country (swamps, caves, deserted mines and buildings), and avoid rocky crevices and ledges.

2. Watch where you step, sit, and reach. Be careful walking over rocks and fallen logs, and don't reach into holes or bushes. Stay on clear paths when possible. Check your sleeping bag, clothing, and boots before using them.

3. Wear knee-high leather boots, long pants, and long-sleeved shirts when you are in snake country.

4. The night belongs to the snakes. Stay in camp after sundown.

5. Don't pick up any snake, even a dead one. Remember, decapitated snakes can bite.

Plant Dermatitis

PRIMARY IRRITANT PLANTS

THORNS, BRISTLES, HAIRS, AND CHEMICALS

There are several groups of plants whose juices contain acids, detergents, and other irritating chemicals that can cause skin irritation. This is not an allergic rash; anyone exposed to the juices of these plants will develop some degree of redness, burning, and itching, depending on the area of the body exposed to the plant. The skin is thick and hard on the palms and soles and resistant to irritation. The skin on the face, neck, chest, and tops of the hands and feet is thinner and more sensitive to these plants.

Crown-of-thorns, snow-on-the-mountain, candelabra cactus, milk buds, and other members of the spurge family have a milky white sap that causes a weepy, red, blistery rash. Marsh marigolds, anemones, buttercups, and other members of the buttercup family have a highly irritant oil in their sap that can cause a similar rash.

Nettles have stinging hairs on their leaves that poke into the skin and inject a stream of irritating chemicals that incite a small riot on the skin surface, causing a hivelike reaction. The skin burns and itches intensely for about an hour and remains red for a variable period.

Contact with the mustard seed plant and radishes can lead to blisters.

Symptom Chart: Plant Dermatitis

Is rash burning and red?	**YES**	Evaluate and treat for exposure to nettles and similar plants, pp. 122–23
NO		
Is rash red and itchy but without blisters?	**YES**	Evaluate and treat for minor poison ivy dermatitis, pp. 125–26
NO		
Is rash blistered and itchy, possibly covering large area of skin?	**YES**	Evaluate and treat for severe poison ivy dermatitis, pp. 125–26

TREATMENT

Primary irritant dermatitis is short-lived. Wash the exposed area with soap and water to remove irritant chemicals. Later you can apply cold Burow's solution compresses and take an antihistamine as needed to control itching.

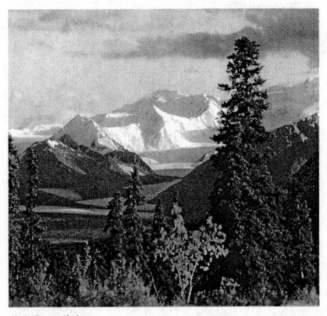

Alaska Range, Alaska

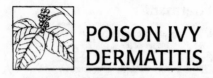

POISON IVY
DERMATITIS

GEOGRAPHICAL DISTRIBUTION

Poison ivy, poison oak, or poison sumac grow in all of the lower 48 states. Poison ivy generally is found east of the Rockies, poison oak west of the Rockies, and poison sumac in the Southeast. Poison ivy is rarely found at elevations above 4,000 feet (1,219 m) or in deserts or rain forests, but it grows exuberantly along cool streams and lake shores. It often blankets sun-drenched hillsides but is found only in isolated patches in cool, dry climates. It grows as a deciduous shrub up to 6 feet (1.8 m) in height or as a small tree or vine. Its shiny leaves are arranged in groups of three ("leaves of three, beware of me") and turn flaming red or reddish violet in late summer or early fall.

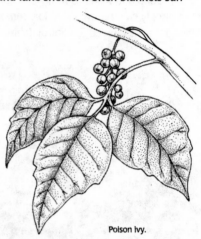

Poison ivy.

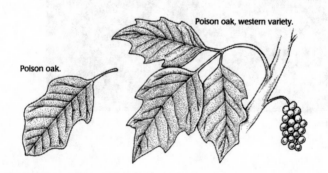

Poison oak, western variety.

Poison oak.

SUSCEPTIBILITY

You may have nothing to fear from poison ivy. About 50 percent of American adults are immune to it. Another 35 percent are "subclinically sensitive;" they are resistant to poison ivy until middle age, when they suddenly break out in a severe rash after

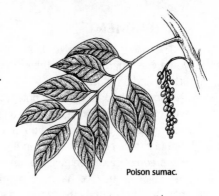

Poison sumac.

rubbing against the broken leaves or stems of the plant. About 15 percent of the population seems to have a natural tolerance to poison ivy.

No one develops a poison ivy rash the first time she touches the plant. First the immune system has to be sensitized to *urushiol*, the oil responsible for the reaction. Then, on subsequent exposures, the body recognizes the oil as a foreign substance and mounts an intense inflammatory response in an effort to destroy it. Repeat exposure maintains the allergic state, but the severity of the allergic reaction tends to diminish with time. A severe bout of poison ivy dermatitis can actually render a person immune to the oil for a period of time.

SIGNS AND SYMPTOMS

Once the sap of the poison ivy plant touches your skin, you become an allergic time bomb if you are sensitive to it. If the resin isn't washed off within an hour or so, you can expect to break out in a rash in 24 to 48 hours. Any area that comes into contact with the resin will react, except the mucous membranes, such as the lips, mouth, and inside of the nose.

The rash starts off as red, swollen lines or patches, with a few small fluid-filled blisters. As the reaction intensifies, the blisters become larger and then break down and weep. The whole area becomes covered with an oozing, scaling crust. (The fluid inside the blisters doesn't contain urushiol, so it can't spread the rash.)

The poison ivy rash is one of the itchiest known to man, and it's almost impossible to resist the temptation to scratch it. But scratching introduces bacteria into the open sores, and secondary bacterial infection is a common problem.

TREATMENT

The rash usually resolves in about 14 days, no matter what you do. But there are a few things that can ease the intense itching and promote healing.

Corticosteroids, a group of potent anti-inflammatory drugs, are your best weapon against poison ivy dermatitis, but only if they are given early. An injection of a high-potency cortico-steroid can be curative if given in the first 24 hours. After that, oral prednisone can be given to tame the inflammation if the rash involves the face, hands, or genitals, or involves more than 30 percent of the body surface area. The usual recommendation for adults is 1 to 2 mg/kg/day tapered over 10 to 20 days.

Topical corticosteroids aren't nearly as effective, although high-potency fluorinated steroids help if used before blisters appear. They also are useful in treating the flare-up of itching that is sometimes seen late in the healing phase.

And don't forget these ancillary measures.

- Cool Burow's solution compresses relieve the itching and accelerate drying. Do this for 15 minutes three to four times a day.

- Calamine also helps relieve itching and promotes drying. Apply a layer of it after each session with the cold compresses.

- If large areas of skin are involved, oatmeal baths are helpful. Add a cup of Aveeno oatmeal to the tub, and soak in it for 15 minutes two or three times a day.

- Oral antihistamines relieve itching, but antihistamine lotions don't help. Anesthetic sprays and lotions not only don't help, they may actually sensitize the skin and aggravate the rash.

PREVENTION

- Familiarize yourself with the plant and avoid it.

- If you are very sensitive to poison ivy, a barrier cream (IvyBlock, Stokogard Outdoor Cream, Hollister Moisture Barrier, and Hydropel Moisture Barrier) can give you some protection.

- If you *do* come into contact with the plant, wash it off with soap and water immediately. Then wash all contaminated clothing and equipment. Water deactivates urushiol, and you can prevent or minimize your reaction to it if you wash it off your skin within two hours, although it's best to wash as soon as possible.

Infectious Diarrhea and Field Water Disinfection

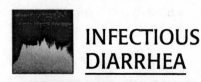 ## INFECTIOUS DIARRHEA

GIARDIASIS, a.k.a. "BACKPACKER'S DIARRHEA"

You may find it hard to believe that a pristine stream high up in the High Sierra, the Rockies, or the Adirondacks could be fouled with disease-causing parasites, but most of them are. Here's how it happens: *Giardia lamblia*, a protozoan parasite, is carried in the small intestine of infected humans, beavers, and other animals in the mature *(trophozoite)* form. Periodically, these trophozoites turn into cysts, split in two, and pass out in the stool. These cysts may lie around on the ground or in a lake or stream for two or three months before they are ingested by an unsuspecting animal or human. As the cysts pass through their host's stomach, they mature into the active trophozoite form. The trophozoites multiply manyfold, until the walls of the upper small intestine are blanketed with *Giardia*, which cause diarrhea. Some of the trophozoites are transformed into cysts, pass out in the stool, and start the cycle again.

Symptoms: Most people who become infected have no symptoms. They become asymptomatic carriers. Other people, after an incubation period of one to three weeks, will experience explosive, watery diarrhea, abdominal cramps, fever, vomiting, and foul flatus. Most victims have milder, lingering diarrhea alternating with soft stools and constipation, bloating, belching, burning indigestion, and nausea. *Giardia* usually runs its course within a few weeks whether it's treated or not. But

Symptom Chart: Infectious Diarrhea

Is patient thirsty with slightly dry tongue after onset of diarrhea? **YES**	Treat for diarrhea with mild dehydration, p. 129
NO	
Is patient very thirsty, tired, with elevated pulse rate after onset of diarrhea? **YES**	Treat for diarrhea with moderate dehydration, p. 129
NO	
Is patient experiencing chills, fever, and/or blood in stools after onset of diarrhea? **YES**	Evaluate and treat for severe diarrhea, pp. 128–29

you'll recover faster and stop shedding cysts a lot sooner if you take a course of an appropriate antibiotic (see your doctor).

TREATMENT

The key to surviving diarrhea, whether it's caused by a virus, bacteria, or *Giardia*, is to avoid dehydration. Symptoms of mild dehydration include slightly increased thirst, slightly dry tongue and lips, and slightly decreased urine output. Moderate dehydration causes moderately increased thirst, increased pulse rate, listlessness, and dry tongue and lips. Take frequent sips of water, juice, weak tea, or other clear liquids. If your fluid losses are large, you'll need to drink 4 to 5 quarts (4 to 5 L) of fluid every 24 hours. Sweetened drinks are especially good because sugar increases the absorption of water by the bowel. Staples such as bananas, cereals, lentils, and potatoes are good sources of calories and nutrients. Avoid caffeine, alcohol, high-fiber foods, and fatty foods.

If you are at a well-supplied base camp, you can mix a batch of the oral rehydration solution recommended by the World Health Organization. To 1 liter of potable water add 1 cup (237 mL) of orange juice, 4 teaspoons (20 mL) of sugar, 1 teaspoon (5 mL) of baking powder, and ¾ teaspoon (3.8 mL) of salt. Drink 30 to 50 mL/kg over the next few hours if you are mildly dehydrated, 100 mL/kg if you are moderately dehydrated.

If you continue to have severe diarrhea (more than 10 stools a day), persistent vomiting, fever, or blood and mucous in the stool, you need to get to a hospital. Blood and mucous suggest the possibility of colitis or a bacterial infection, especially if you have fever and chills.

PREVENTION

Giardia and other microbes that cause infectious diarrhea are transmitted by the fecal-oral route. Control their spread by observing these rules of personal hygiene in the wild.

- Bury human waste 12 inches (30 cm) deep at least 100 yards (91 m) from the nearest water.

- Do not defecate within 40 yards (37 m) of a lake shore or stream runoff.

- Wash your hands after each bowel movement.

- Do not prepare food if you have diarrhea.

- Rinse cooking utensils and dishes in chlorinated water.

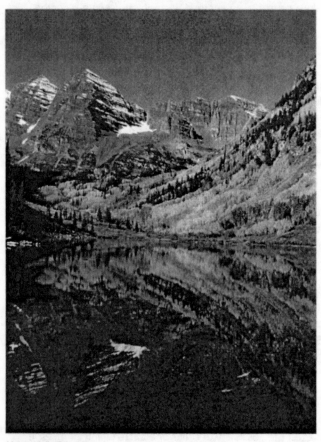

Maroon Bells, Colorado

WATER DISINFECTION

The aim in disinfecting water is to remove or destroy the harmful microorganisms in it. What you want is *potable water*, water that's safe to drink. It may have a few microorganisms in it but not any more than your body can easily fight off.

You can disinfect water using physical or chemical methods.

PHYSICAL METHODS

Sedimentation: The disinfection process will be more effective if you start with the clearest water available. Cloudy, muddy water is a suspension of silt and clay particles and organic debris that may be contaminated with bacteria and parasitic cysts. You can rely on sedimentation to separate out the bigger particles simply by allowing the water to sit for an hour or more. These large particles will settle on the bottom of the container, and you can decant the clear water into another container.

Coagulation-flocculation: Small particles and chemicals in the decanted water will remain suspended in the decanted water, but you can precipitate them out. Add ⅛ to ¼ teaspoon (0.6–1.3 mL) of *alum* (aluminum sulfate) per gallon (4 L) of water, stir for five minutes, and allow the suspension to settle for an hour before you decant it or pour it through a coffee filter or fine-weave cloth. Then disinfect the water using heat or chemical means. If you don't have alum, you can use baking powder (3 oz. per 5 gal. of water/89 mL per 19 L), baking soda (1 oz. per 5 gal. of water/29.6 mg per 19 L), charcoal from a wood fire (2 lb. per 5 gal. of water/0.9 kg per 19 L), or fine white ash from a wood fire (2 oz. per 5 gal. of water/59 mL per 19 L).

Filters: Mechanical water filters consist of a screen with pore sizes as small as 0.2 microns and an activated charcoal element. Micropore filters will remove *Giardia* cysts and most bacteria, but not viruses, so the water will have to be either boiled or chemically treated before it is used. Charcoal filters containing granular activated charcoal (GAC) remove bad tastes and odors from water by adsorbing dissolved chemicals. GAC adsorbs some, but not all, viruses and bacteria, so it cannot be relied upon to disinfect water. It's most useful for removing chlorine and iodine from water after chemical disinfection.

Heat: If you have ample fuel, the simplest way to disinfect water is to bring it to a boil. No additional heating time is required at high altitudes.

If you melt snow or ice for drinking water, bring it to a boil just as you would any other water. It's probably just as contaminated as the surface water in the area.

CHEMICAL METHODS

Giardia, viruses, and bacteria can all be killed by chemical disinfection with *halogens* (iodine or chlorine). Halogens oxidize the essential cell structures of microorganisms when they are in contact with them in high enough concentration for a sufficient period of time.

Contact time and concentration of halogen are inversely related. The greater the concentration of halogen, the less time is necessary to destroy microorganisms. Conversely, the longer the contact time, the lower the concentration of halogen necessary to disinfect the water. For example, if you double the concentration of halogen, the water will be disinfected in half the time. Or you can halve the concentration of halogen if you simply double the contact time.

The third factor influencing the disinfection reaction is water temperature. When disinfecting cold water, either the contact time or the concentration of halogen has to be doubled to insure disinfection.

Halogens in high concentrations impart a bad taste to water. The taste of halogen-treated water can be improved by

- using less halogen and increasing the contact time
- filtering the water with granular activated charcoal after the contact time
- adding flavoring to the water after the contact time
- using a zinc brush, ascorbic acid (vitamin C), or sodium thiosulfate

HALOGEN DOSES AND TECHNIQUES* (ALL DOSES ADDED TO 1 QT. OR 1 L OF WATER)

Iodination Techniques	Amount for 4 ppm	Amount for 8 ppm
iodine tablets (tetraglycine hydroperiodide; EDWGT, Potable Aqua, Globaline)	½ tab	1 tab
Solutions		
2% iodine (tincture)	5 drops	10 drops
10% povidone-iodine solution (Betadine)	8 drops	16 drops
saturated iodine crystals in water (Polar Pure)	13 mL	26 mL
saturated iodine crystals in alcohol	0.1 mL for 5 ppm	0.2 mL for 10 ppm
Chlorination		
Halazone tablets	2 tabs	4 tabs
household bleach	2 drops	4 drops

* Reprinted with permission from the *Wilderness Medical Society Practice Guidelines for Wilderness Emergency Care,* Wilderness Medical Society, 2001.

Concentration of Halogen	Contact Time in Minutes at Various Water Temperatures		
	41°F (5°C)	59°F (15°C)	86°F (30°C)
2 ppm	240	180	60
4 ppm	180	60	45
8 ppm	60	30	15

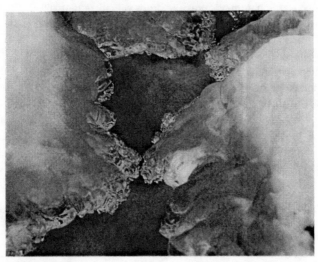

Boulder Creek, Colorado

High-Altitude Illness

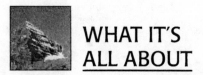

WHAT IT'S ALL ABOUT

You don't have to go to the Himalaya to get high-altitude illness. Most people who rapidly ascend above 8,000 feet (2,400 m) develop one or more symptoms of acute mountain sickness. This and the other forms of high-altitude illness can make any high-country trek not only unpleasant but dangerous as well.

Here's the problem: Oxygen is the fuel that drives your metabolic machinery. But the machinery starts to sputter when you climb over 4,900 feet (1,500 m) above sea level and the air gets thinner. As the barometric pressure drops with increasing altitude, oxygen molecules spread out; there are fewer of them in each breath that you take, a condition known as *hypoxia*. The oxygen content of the blood drops, so less oxygen is delivered to the tissues. But an increase in the rate and depth of breathing, increased heart rate, and other physiological adaptations allow the body to acclimatize to the thinner air.

Symptom Chart: High-Altitude Illness

Does patient exhibit chest congestion; pink, frothy sputum; bluish lips and fingernail beds; and rapid pulse and breathing?	**YES** ▶	Evaluate and treat for severe high-altitude pulmonary edema, p. 139
NO ⬇		
Does patient exhibit dry cough, loss of stamina, and increased weakness?	**YES** ▶	Evaluate and treat for mild high-altitude pulmonary edema, p. 139
NO ⬇		
Does patient exhibit loss of coordination, staggering gait, confusion, and stupor?	**YES** ▶	Evaluate and treat for high-altitude cerebral edema, p. 139
NO ⬇		
Does patient experience headache, dizziness, loss of appetite, and fatigue a few hours after ascent to high altitude, possibly with displays of irritability, nausea, vomiting, or swelling in hands and feet?	**YES** ▶	Evaluate and treat for mountain sickness, pp. 136–37

Hypoxia progressively reduces your ability to perform muscular work or exercise as you ascend to higher altitudes. You have to breathe harder just to satisfy your body's resting requirements for oxygen. Breathing itself becomes a chore. You also develop *periodic breathing*—waxing and waning cycles of heavy and light breathing interspersed with intervals of no breathing. This increased work of breathing and periodic breathing wreak havoc on the sleep cycle. Difficulty falling asleep, frequent awakening, and bizarre dreams are common at higher altitudes.

ACUTE MOUNTAIN SICKNESS

TOO HIGH, TOO FAST

Acute mountain sickness (AMS) is common in unacclimated people who rapidly ascend to 6,500 feet (2,000 m) or higher. Whether or not you get AMS depends upon how high you ascend, how quickly you make the ascent, how much you exert yourself during and after the ascent, how long you stay at high altitude, and your own individual susceptibility to it.

Hypoxia is the root cause of AMS, but it's the body's reaction to this deficiency of oxygen that causes the symptoms. Researchers believe that insufficient breathing for the conditions, fluid retention, the shift of fluids into the cells, increase in pressure on the brain, and the accumulation of water in the lungs all contribute to the development of acute mountain sickness. Of these, the buildup of pressure on the brain is probably the most important factor.

SYMPTOMS

AMS usually starts one to six hours after the ascent, or after the first night at high altitude, and resembles a hangover. The most prominent symptoms are headache, dizziness, loss of appetite, and fatigue. You may also experience lassitude, sleepiness, a deep inner chill, nausea, vomiting, irritability, shortness of breath on exertion, and swelling of the face, hands, and feet. Loss of coordination, staggering gait, and altered level of consciousness are signs of high-altitude cerebral edema (HACE), discussed below.

TREATMENT

You can stay put, and the symptoms of mild AMS will resolve in one to four days. (Do not go up until your symptoms go down.) Or you can descend 1,600 to 3,300 feet (500–1,000 m) and get better quickly. Supplemental oxygen (at a flow rate of 1 liter/minute) helps, if you have it. Limiting your movements also helps. Aspirin, ibuprofen, or acetaminophen will usually relieve the headache of acute mountain sickness. Promethazine (Phenergan) can be given as a 25 mg suppository every eight hours to control nausea. Salt restriction counteracts the body's tendency to retain fluids at altitude. Acetazolamide increases respiratory drive, which accelerates acclimatization to high altitude, and can be used to prevent and treat AMS. Dexamethasone, a corticosteroid, is also effective in treating AMS. The dose is 4 mg every six hours. A hyperbaric bag can be used to simulate descent.

If symptoms don't resolve despite treatment, the victim needs to descend to a lower altitude. When he starts to stagger, refuses to eat or drink, insists on being left alone, and becomes progressively more confused, disoriented, and lethargic, he is suffering from severe mountain sickness and needs to be led back down the mountain right away.

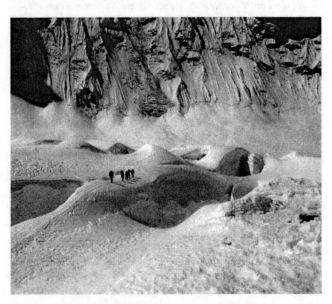

Climbers ascending to Camp 2, Mt. Everest.

PREVENTION

Here are some ways to avoid mountain sickness.

- *Stage your ascent.* Allow yourself time to acclimatize to the thin air at altitude. The key is where you sleep. Your respiratory drive is diminished at night, so that is when your blood oxygen levels fall to their lowest point. Your first camp should be at 8,000 feet (2,400 m) or lower, with subsequent camps at intervals of 1,000 to 2,000 feet (300–600 m). Or you can spend two nights at the same altitude for every 2,000-foot ascent, starting at 10,000 feet (3,000 m). Climb higher during the day; then return to a lower elevation to sleep ("climb high, sleep low").

- *Avoid alcohol and sleeping medications.* Both suppress your respiratory drive, and alcohol increases the hangover effect and causes dehydration. Caffeine and cocoa are beneficial because they stimulate the respiratory drive.

- *Stay well hydrated.* You lose more fluids at high altitudes. If you are not putting out lots of clear urine, you need to drink more fluids.

- *Avoid strenuous exercise* until you are acclimatized. Mild exercise probably aids acclimatization.

- A *high-carbohydrate diet* (greater than 70 percent carbohydrates) started a day or two before your climb will reduce the symptoms of AMS by one-third.

- *Drug prophylaxis.* Acetazolamide will prevent acute mountain sickness in most cases. If you are forced to climb rapidly to a sleeping altitude greater than 9,000 feet (2,700 m), start taking acetazolamide, 125 mg twice a day, 24 hours before you start your ascent. You should also take it if you have a history of AMS. *Warning*: Do not use acetazolamide if you are pregnant or allergic to sulfa. If you cannot take acetazolamide or are forced to ascend rapidly to very high altitude (over 14,000 feet, or 4,250 meters), take dexamethasone 4 mg by mouth every six hours, starting two to four hours before you begin your ascent.

HIGH-ALTITUDE CEREBRAL EDEMA

High-altitude cerebral edema (HACE), the severest form of AMS, is progressive deterioration of neurologic function due to brain swelling. The hallmarks are loss of coordination, staggering gait, confusion, and stupor. Most HACE victims also have HAPE (high-altitude pulmonary edema; see below), and some develop headache, nausea, vomiting, hallucinations, paralysis, and abnormal eye movements. If untreated, the victim may lapse into coma and die.

HACE is treated by immediate descent to a lower elevation and with oxygen and dexamethasone.

HIGH-ALTITUDE PULMONARY EDEMA

After rapid ascent to high altitude, the blood vessels supplying the lungs sometimes become "leaky," and the lungs become engorged with fluid. This is called high-altitude pulmonary edema (HAPE). It is much more common in young men and usually develops within the first two to four days after ascending to altitude, often during the second night.

Symptoms: The first signs of HAPE are a dry cough, fatigue, shortness of breath on exertion, weakness, and decreased stamina. Severe HAPE is marked by profound weakness, bluish discoloration of the lips and nails, shortness of breath at rest, chest congestion, rapid pulse and respiratory rates, and altered consciousness. Coma and pink, frothy sputum are harbingers of death.

Treatment: HAPE is the most common cause of death at high altitude, so it must be recognized while it is still in the mild stage and treated by heading down the hill pronto. A descent of 1,600 to 3,300 feet (500–1,000 m) may be lifesaving. A hyperbaric bag or oxygen will help if rapid descent is impossible.

Prevention: Measures that help to prevent acute mountain sickness also help to prevent HAPE. Nifedipine, 20 mg by mouth every eight hours while ascending and for three additional days at altitude, is an effective prophylactic drug, as is acetazolamide.

Foot Care in the Wild

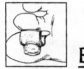

BLISTERS

CAUSES

Most blisters are caused by new or poorly fitting boots. They usually develop over the toes, the front of the foot, and the heel, where the skin is thick and tough and bound down to the underlying bone. As your foot slides back and forth inside your boot, shearing forces produce small clefts within the skin. Fluid then flows into these clefts and, voilà, you have a blister.

If your boots are too loose in the instep, you will get "downhill blisters" on your toes and the front of your feet as your foot slides forward while hiking downhill. You may get "uphill blisters" on the heel or over the Achilles tendon while climbing steep trails.

You can always count on your feet getting hot and moist when you hike on a warm spring or fall day, and a hot, slightly moist foot is a blister waiting to happen. A thin layer of moisture causes your socks to adhere more tightly to your skin and increases friction within the skin. When your feet are soaked or dry, there is less friction between socks and feet, and less risk of blistering.

Walking on blistered feet is about as much fun as walking barefoot across a bed of hot coals. One well-placed blister can severely reduce your mobility and put a real crimp in your hiking style. A neglected or improperly treated blister can become ulcerated and infected and spawn a rapidly spreading skin infection called *cellulitis*, or even *sepsis* (blood poisoning).

Symptom Chart: Foot Problems

Does foot have red, tender area(s) that feels hot but with no blistering? **YES** →	Evaluate and treat for hot spot, p. 141		
NO ↓			
Does foot have red, tender area(s) with blisters? **YES** →	Is blister intact? **YES** →	Evaluate and treat for intact blisters, pp. 141–42	
NO ↓	**NO** ↓		
	Evaluate and treat for torn blisters, p. 141		
Are there small areas of tough dry skin on foot? **YES** →	Is pain between fourth and fifth toe? **YES** →	Evaluate and treat for soft corns, p. 144	
NO ↓	**NO** ↓		
	Evaluate and treat for hard corns, p. 144		
Is fleshy area at edge of big toe red, inflamed, and painful? **YES** →	Evaluate and treat for ingrown toenail, p. 144		
NO ↓			
Is there itching between toes with redness and scaling? **YES** →	Evaluate and treat for athlete's foot, p. 145		

TREATMENT

A hot spot is a red, tender area, an incipient blister. Never ignore a hot spot: cover it immediately with a bandage, a piece of smooth tape, or a hydrogel dressing.

If the roof of the blister is torn, use scissors to remove the dead skin. Then cleanse it with antiseptic solution or soapy water, and cover it with antibiotic ointment and a bandage twice daily until it heals.

If the roof of the blister is nearly intact, don't remove it. It serves as a biological dressing, and the blister will heal faster if its roof reattaches to its base. Cleanse the blister; then apply a layer of antibiotic ointment and cover it with a bandage or a strip of tape. If you have a hydrogel dressing, apply it to the blister and cover with the adhesive knit bandage provided. Moisten the hydrogel dressing through the bandage several times a day, and leave it in place until the blister heals. If you don't have a hydrogel dressing, cover the blister with gauze or felt, secure it with tape or moleskin, and apply a layer of petrolatum over the tape or moleskin to decrease friction. (The tape or moleskin will adhere better if you first apply benzoin to the skin around the blister.) Check the wound in three days. Remove any dead skin, and reapply the bandage for three more days.

If the blister is intact, drain it. First cleanse the area with antiseptic solution or soapy water. Then puncture the edge of the blister with a sterile needle or a pin that has been sterilized in an open flame. Gently press on the blister to express the fluid; then apply antibiotic ointment and a bandage. Puncture the blister three times within the first 24 hours or once 24 to 36 hours after the blister forms.

If the blister starts to drain cloudy fluid or pus, the surrounding skin becomes red and tender, or you see red streaks extending up your foot, infection has set in. *Never take a foot infection lightly!* Stay off your feet, keep the infected foot elevated above heart level, and soak it in warm, soapy, water every 4 hours. Take cefadroxil, 500 mg every 12 hours. If the infection doesn't start to resolve within 36 hours, head home and see a physician *immediately*, especially if you develop fever or chills.

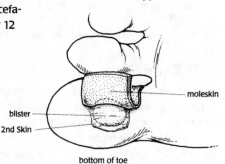

bottom of toe

Cleanse blister with soap and water, then apply 2nd Skin and a layer of moleskin.

PREVENTION

An ounce of prevention is worth a pound of cure, and the best way to prevent blisters is by reducing friction between your boots and your feet. Here's how.

- Make sure your boots fit well. Shop for a new pair in the afternoon, when your feet are slightly swollen, and wear the socks that you plan to wear with the boots. Walk around in them for a few minutes to see if they are comfortable, and make sure that there is a thumb's width of space between the tip of the longest toe and the end of the boot.

- Break new shoes in gradually by wearing them for a couple of hours the first day then an additional hour each day thereafter until they are supple and fit your feet perfectly.

- If there are any loose or tight areas in either boot after you have worn them for a few days, you can work the leather to make it more supple or apply a shoe insert or pad to tighten loose areas.

- Wear a combination of socks that will limit moisture and friction (see Sock Talk, page 145).

- Apply foot powder liberally at least twice a day. Foot powder absorbs moisture and reduces friction by keeping your feet dry. Drysol (20 percent aluminum chloride hexahydrate) and other antiperspirants inhibit sweating. If you don't have an antiperspirant in your pack, boil a couple of tea bags in a pint of water for 15 minutes, add the tea to 2 quarts (2 L) of cool water, and soak your feet in the solution for 20 minutes every night. Tannic acid in the tea will keep your feet dry and smelling like roses.

- Keep blister-prone areas covered with tape, moleskin, or petrolatum, and apply benzoin or alum powder to these areas to toughen the skin.

- Toughen up your feet and tune up your muscles and your cardiovascular system a few weeks before your wilderness trek by taking progressively longer hikes in the boots you plan to wear during your sojourn in the wild.

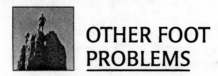

OTHER FOOT PROBLEMS

CORNS AND CALLUSES

Tight-fitting shoes or deformed feet or toes can produce calluses—thickening of the tough layer of dead cells on the surface of the skin. Calluses are protective, but when they become too thick, they are pushed inward and become hard corns over bony protuberances, such as over the top of the fourth toe. Soft corns are painful little volcano-shaped calluses between your fourth and fifth toes. They are painful because the skin at the bottom of these craters is perpetually bathed in perspiration, which causes it to become very thin and sensitive to pressure.

Treatment: Pare the callus or corn with a scalpel or callus file, and cover it with a pad. A wisp of cotton between the toes soaks up perspiration and decreases pressure on the skin. Wider boots will help too.

INGROWN TOENAILS

Tight boots can also cause ingrown toenails. The thick, rigid edge of the nail of the big toe digs into the adjoining skin, producing redness, irritation, swelling, and "weeping" as the inflamed skin secretes fluid.

Treatment: First, cut a V in the middle of the nail to make it more flexible. Then fold a small sheet of aluminum foil until it's the size of a match head and insert it under the corner of the nail where it's digging into the skin. Place a wisp of cotton along the nail to keep the area dry, and keep the foot elevated as much as possible.

If these conservative measures don't work or infection develops, seek medical attention.

ATHLETE'S FOOT

After a few days on the trail, your feet can get downright grungy with accumulated sweat. The heat and moisture inside your boots encourage growth of *Trichophyton*, *Microsporum*, and other fungi that causes *athlete's foot*. Scaling, red, intensely itchy areas, with vesicles and fissuring between the toes, are characteristic of this condition.

Treatment: The key to prevention and cure is to eliminate heat and perspiration. Wear shoes and light cotton socks that allow adequate ventilation. Wash and gently dry the feet every day, if possible, and apply clotrimazole (Lotrimin) cream or tolnaftate (Tinactin) liquid to infected areas twice daily. Sprinkle an antifungal powder containing tolnaftate or undecylenic acid between the toes and into the socks every morning. The powder will soak up moisture and destroy the fungus before it can establish a toehold on your feet.

SOCK TALK

When you're packing your gear, don't just reach blindly into your drawer for a pair of socks to wear with your hiking boots. Pack several pairs, including thin, 100 percent acrylic socks to wear as an inner layer, thicker cotton or wool socks (depending on the season) to wear as an outer layer, or some of the new "double-layered" socks. When you wear two or three pairs of socks, movement occurs mostly between the layers of socks rather than between your sock and skin.

Acrylic socks hold their shape and wear better than cotton socks, dry quickly, and wick moisture away from the skin. They are also thinner over the top of the foot, which allows for better air circulation. If you have bunions or hammer toes, wear socks with extra cushioning in the toes.

Fit is important too. Your socks should be higher than your boot tops and loose enough that they don't bunch up or wrinkle, but not so tight that they pinch your toes. Always carry extra socks on your person in case your feet get wet.

Wilderness Evacuation

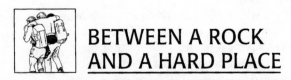

BETWEEN A ROCK
AND A HARD PLACE

Jim knew they were in trouble even before Dan broke his ankle. They had spent the morning hiking in the high country near Yellowstone Park, but a furious early-season snowstorm swept into the area at midday and high winds and poor visibility forced them to call it quits and head back to camp. They had hiked only a few hundred yards down the trail when Dan lost his footing on a snow-slicked rock and went airborne. He came down with all of his weight on his right ankle, and his lower tibia snapped with a loud "crack," a sound Jim mistook for a breaking pine bough until he looked up and saw Dan writhing in the snow. His partner's right ankle was grotesquely deformed, and a blood stain was spreading across his pant leg.

Jim set and splinted Dan's fractured ankle, then paused to consider his options. It would be dark in a couple of hours, and the drifting snow had almost obliterated the trail. Dan needed urgent medical attention, but the trailhead was a five-hour hike down the mountain in good conditions. There was no way he could carry him that far on his back in a snowstorm. Heck, he'd be lucky if he could lug him the 2 miles back to camp before dark!

What would you do if you were in Jim's position? Would you make a heroic effort to carry Dan out of the wilderness in a blizzard? Would you try to get him back to camp? Or would you find shelter, settle in for the night, and reassess the situation in the morning?

In this scenario, the last option is the most prudent one, although an argument could be made for carrying your injured buddy back to camp if you felt up to the task and were familiar with one-rescuer evacuation techniques. Any attempt to carry him out of the woods that afternoon would end in tragedy.

EVACUATION GUIDELINES

There is no formula that will tell you precisely what to do in every situation, but you can use the following guidelines to map out a strategy for dealing with any wilderness evacuation problem.

- Anyone with a minor injury or an upper extremity injury should be able to walk back to camp or to the trailhead under her own power.

- Most people with leg or foot injuries can be carried out. Anyone with multiple fractures or spinal, chest, or abdominal injuries may need to be evacuated by helicopter.

- A strong, fit person may be able to carry an injured adult on his back for a mile or two, but two or more people will be needed for longer transports, especially over rugged terrain.

- Never leave an unconscious, confused, or otherwise helpless person unattended.

- In remote, mountainous areas, self-evacuation is often faster than sending a messenger and waiting for help to arrive.

- Never set out on an evacuation at night or in severe weather.

- Don't create additional victims by placing yourself or others in a dangerous position during a medical evacuation.

If you elect to send for help, dispatch the fittest member of the group with a map showing your location, trails, natural landmarks, and the best route to the trailhead, and a note specifying the number of victims, their ages, the nature of their injuries, their condition, treatment given, supplies needed, and the urgency of the situation. Then erect a shelter and mark it so that it will be easily visible to rescuers. Smoke can be seen from the ground or air, and a large X laid out with sticks or stones in an open field or meadow will signal aircraft that you need medical assistance.

Generally, the wisest course is to wait with the victim while someone goes for help, but impending bad weather, inadequate clothing or shelter, dwindling food and water supplies, or worsening of the victim's condition may force your hand.

RESCUE CARRIES

ONE-RESCUER CARRIES

Carrying your partner out of the woods will seem like the Twelve Labors of Hercules if you don't go about it the right way. After you have stabilized the victim as well as you can (see pages 12–14), you'll need to devise a way to convey her out of the woods. If you are the lone rescuer, you can use one of these one-rescuer carries.

Backpack carry: Cut leg holes in the bottom of a large backpack, have the injured person climb into it, and then hoist it onto your back.

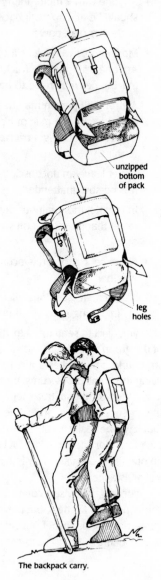

unzipped bottom of pack

leg holes

The backpack carry.

Rope seat: Pass a long, 1-inch (2.5 cm) rope or strap over the victim's head, and pull the ends under his armpits and across his chest. Then lift him onto your back piggyback fashion and pull the rope ends over your shoulders, under your arms, back between his legs, and then around his upper thighs. Take up the slack; then tie the ends across your waist.

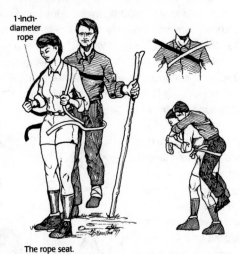

1-inch-diameter rope

The rope seat.

Split-coil carry: Coil a lengthy piece of rope, and fix it at one point with a knot. Divide the coiled rope into two equal loops, and have the victim step into the loops and pull them up snug against his crotch with the fixed segment in front. Then have him stand on a stump or rock while you back up to him, place your arms through the free ends of the loops, and hoist him onto your back.

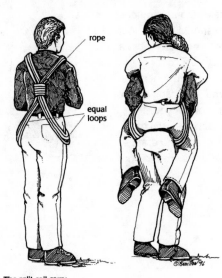

rope

equal loops

The split-coil carry.

TWO-RESCUER CARRIES

Four-hand seat: The rescuers stand facing each other and form a seat for the victim by interlocking hands as follows: each rescuer grasps his right wrist with his left hand and then grasps the other rescuer's left wrist with his right hand palm down.

Pole carry: This technique requires two heavy backpacks or rucksacks, and rescuers of near equal stature. First find a sturdy, 5- to 6-foot-long (1.5–2 m) tree limb and trim off the branches. Next don your backpacks, stand side by side, and pass each end of the tree limb behind the pack and rest it on the hip belt. Then pad the limb, and have the victim sit on it and drape his arms around you and the other rescuer for support.

Coiled-rope seat: Stand shoulder to shoulder with your fellow rescuer, pass a large coiled rope around your necks, and let it hang down in front of you. The victim then sits on the rope and drapes his arms around your shoulders.

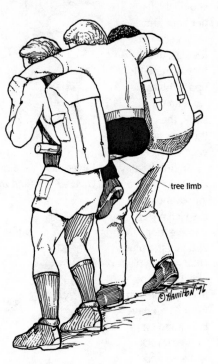

tree limb

The pole carry.

LITTERS

Single- or two-rescuer techniques are appropriate for people with relatively minor injuries or illnesses, but you will have to use a litter to evacuate anyone who is unconscious or has difficulty breathing, a serious chest or abdominal injury, or fractures of the pelvis, hip, or femur. You will need at least six rescuers to carry the patient and litter a short distance and twelve or more for an evacuation over a greater distance.

Before you start out, pad the litter so that the injured person doesn't get bedsores. Give her something to eat and drink, and offer her an analgesic. Make sure that she is secured to the litter and insulated against the cold. Check her condition whenever you stop to rest, and make sure that her bandages haven't soaked through and her splints haven't loosened. Do whatever you can to buck up her spirits.

These litters are serviceable and easy to construct.

POLE LITTER

Select two straight tree limbs or poles about 7 feet (2 m) long and lay them on the ground about 18 inches (46 cm) apart. Then tie cross supports to the limbs at 10- to 12-inch (25–30 cm) intervals.

SLEEPING BAG LITTER

Spread a sleeping bag (or a blanket or tarp) on the ground, and align the poles or tree limbs on it lengthwise, about 15 inches (38 cm) apart. Lash cross supports across the poles about 6 inches (15 cm) from each end, and then fold the sides of the bag over the poles. The victim's weight will keep the bag from slipping between the poles.

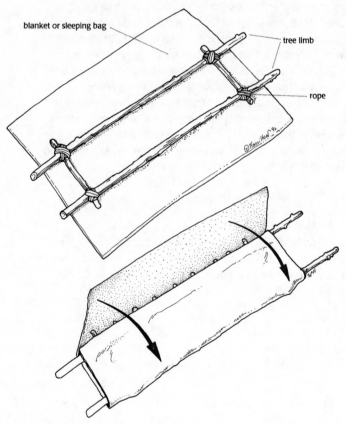

The sleeping bag litter.

POLE-AND-ROPE LITTER

Make a frame as described for the sleeping bag litter; then tie one end of a rope to one corner of the frame. Now loop the rope around one pole 8 to 10 times, leaving enough slack in each loop so that it can be pulled to the midpoint between the two poles, and tie it to the other corner. Then repeat the process on the other side, but this time pass the free end of the rope through the loops you just created so that they interlock. When you are done, pull the rope taut to create a firm rope mattress.

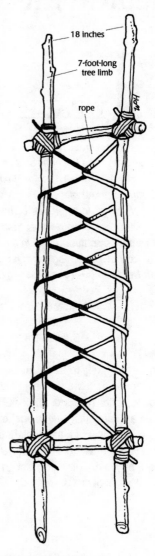

18 inches

7-foot-long tree limb

rope

The pole-and-rope litter.

The Wilderness Medical Kit

WHAT TO TAKE

*Bayley carried a small bottle of spirits for healing,
sustaining and fortifying uses, in case of encounters with
triangular headed snakes, bears, Indians, mountain
rams, noxious night airs, snow storms, etc.; and in case
of vertigo and difficult breathing at great heights, together with broken bones, flesh wounds, skin erosions,
abrasions, contusions. For in prudence, is it not well to realize that "something might happen," and well to have a
helpful spirit—a guardian angel in a bottle ever near?*

—John Muir, from the account of his 1875
ascent of Mount Whitney printed in
the San Francisco *Daily Evening Bulletin*

You're not likely to have any difficulties with Indians when
you're on the trail, but you just might have to deal with a broken bone, a flesh wound, "difficult breathing at great heights,"
or even a "triangular headed snake." You'd be wise to pack not
a bottle of spirits but a lightweight but comprehensive medical
kit that you can use to treat a variety of injuries and illnesses.
You can buy everything you'll need at your local drugstore; or-
ganize it as follows.

WOUND CARE MATERIALS

bar soap

antiseptic solution, 2 oz. bottle

antibiotic ointment, 1 oz. tube; apply a small amount to wound before bandaging (e.g., Neosporin, Bacitracin)

4 Adaptic dressings, 3 x 3in.; nonadherent mesh dressings that prevent bandage from sticking to wound

6 sterile dressing pads, 4 x 4 in.; four-ply pads with wicking action that absorbs blood and other fluids; also good for cleaning wounds

2 Kerlix or Kling roll bandages, 4 in. x 5 yd.; stretchy gauze rolls for bandaging and securing splints

2 Surgipads, 8 x 10 in., or ABD pads, 8 x 8 in.; use to apply pressure to large, bleeding wounds and to cover burns

1 roll waterproof adhesive tape, 1 in. x 5 yd.

4 Bioclusive or Tegaderm transparent dressings, 2 x 3 in. or 3 x 3 in.; high-tech dressings that seal out water and dust but not air; ideal for blisters, abrasions, and small cuts that are not bleeding

Spenco 2nd Skin; a hydrogel that's a great dressing for open blisters and burns

10 bandage strips (Band-Aids), 1 x 3 in.

10 skin closure strips, ¼ x 3 in.; can be used to close clean, relatively superficial cuts instead of stitches (deep, jagged lacerations require treatment at a medical facility); try Butterflies (Johnson & Johnson), Steri-Strips (3M), Curistrips (Kendall), or Coverstrip Closures (Beiersdorf)

10 skin closure strips, ½ x 3 in.

compound benzoin tincture, 2 oz.; will increase the staying power of skin closure strips; apply to skin on either side of wound and let dry until sticky. *Warning*: Benzoin is an organic solvent—don't let it come in contact with the wound itself.

latex surgical gloves, 2 pairs

Dressings and bandages should be stored in a watertight plastic container to insure that they don't get wet.

MEDICINES

20 aspirin, acetaminophen, or ibuprofen tablets

10 diphenhydramine (Benadryl) tabs, 25 mg; always have on hand for allergic reactions and to control severe itching

10 Imodium tablets; a nonprescription antidiarrheal

**5 Phenergan (promethazine) suppositories; contains promethazine; use to control vomiting

*10 Tylox tablets; contains oxycodone, a potent narcotic, and acetaminophen; use for severe pain

*10 Duricef (cefadroxil) 500 mg capsules; effective against staph and strep bacteria, and in treating wound and other soft tissue infections and dental infections

**30 acetazolamide 250 mg tablets; for mountain sickness

**16 Decadron 4 mg tablets; for mountain sickness

**26 Nifedipine 20 mg tablets

calamine lotion 4 oz.; dries weeping, itching poison ivy rashes

10 Domeboro tabs; add one or two tablets to a pint of water to make Burow's solution, an astringent solution

hydrocortisone 1 percent cream, 60 g tube

personal medications

* Prescription medications.

** Include only if you are traveling to high altitude (over 8,000 feet, or 2,400 m).

MISCELLANEOUS

2 instant cold packs

2 elastic (Ace) bandages, 3 and 6 in.; good for wrapping
sprains and applying compression to large, bleeding
wounds

bulb irrigating syringe, 60 cc

triangular bandage; large muslin bandage that can be
used as a sling or turban bandage for head wounds,
or to secure splints to fractured extremities

6 large safety pins; use to secure slings and splints, close
large wounds, or to hold the tongue out of the back
of the throat when the jaw is badly broken

2 tongue blades; good temporary splints for fractured
fingers

scissors

tweezers

needlenose pliers

Sam splint; a lightweight, malleable splint for immobilizing
fractures

moleskin

water-purification tablets (Potable Aqua, Globuline,
Halazone)

dental first-aid kit

Index

Numbers in **bold** refer to pages with illustrations